TANTRIC SEX
FOR MEN

TANTRIC SEX FOR MEN

Making Love a Meditation

DIANA RICHARDSON

AND

MICHAEL RICHARDSON

Destiny Books
Rochester, Vermont • Toronto, Canada

Destiny Books
One Park Street
Rochester, Vermont 05767
www.DestinyBooks.com

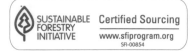

Text stock is SFI certified

Destiny Books is a division of Inner Traditions International

Library of Congress Cataloging-in-Publication Data

Richardson, Diana.
  Tantric sex for men : making love a meditation / Diana Richardson and Michael
Richardson.
     p. cm.
  Includes bibliographical references and index.
  ISBN 978-1-59477-311-2 (pbk.)
  1. Sex instruction for men. 2. Sex instruction—Religious aspects—Tantrism. I.
Richardson, Michael. II. Title.
  HQ36.R524 2010
  613.9'6—dc22

                                                                    2010012680

Printed and bound in the United States by Lake Book Manufacturing, Inc.
The text paper is 100% SFI certified. The Sustainable Forestry Initiative® program
promotes sustainable forest management.

10   9

Text design and layout by Virginia Scott Bowman
This book was typeset in Garamond Premier Pro with Weiss, Gill Sans, and
Helvetica as display typefaces

All Osho quotes printed with permission of Osho International
Artwork prepared by Alfredo Hernando, Madrid, Spain
Author cover photographs by Shobha, Sicily, Italy

Dedicated to Mother Earth

Tantric Inspiration

Even after a lifetime of sexual experience we never reach anywhere near that supreme stage, near that divinity. Why? A man reaches a ripe old age, comes to the end of his life, but he is never free from his lust for sex, from his passion for intercourse. Why? It is because he has never understood nor been told about the art of sex, about the science of sex. He has never considered it; he has never discussed it with the enlightened ones.

OSHO, TRANSCRIBED TEACHINGS,
FROM SEX TO SUPERCONSCIOUSNESS

CONTENTS

Tantric Inspiration

When sex is just an unconscious, mechanical urge in you, it is wrong. Remember, sex is not wrong: just the mechanicalness of it is wrong. If you can bring some light of intelligence into your sexuality, that light will transform it. It will not be sexuality anymore—it will be something totally different, so different that you do not have a word for it.

In the East we have a word for it—Tantra. In the West you don't have a word for it. When sex becomes joined together, is yoked with intelligence, a totally new energy is created—that energy is called Tantra.

OSHO, TRANSCRIBED TEACHINGS,
PHILOSOPHIA PERENNIS

PREFACE

By Michael Richardson

Sex is not what it seems to be. We all have inherited preconceptions and ideas about sex, which are mostly false and form a screen, or barrier, that separates us from the real power of sex. When we look beyond the inherited screen of misunderstanding we discover that sex is completely different from what we generally think it is. Through sexual exploration I personally have discovered the true function of sex, which is to bring more love into the world. Each and every person can be a messenger of love by creating more love and contributing it to the world.

The screen of conditioning—our past experiences and ideas—limits our human sexual expression. After all, what does a man want when he makes love to a woman? What is the ultimate reason for making love? It is not to achieve ejaculation; it is to be loved by the woman.

Woman is the source of love, the mother of love, and I, as a man, am able to tap into that love. For me, love is what it is all about. Being in the here and now, I've discovered that in stillness, including inner stillness during movement, I can tap into or connect with the "garden of love" in woman. And there is nothing more satisfying and touching than seeing a woman radiating, blossoming in love.

I do have hope for humanity. The only hope is for man to find a way through his screen of conditioned sexuality, so that he may come to rest within his male authority. So that he can make peace with woman and make love to her body, heart, and soul.

INTRODUCTION

There are a great many books about sex offering a range of techniques best described as the "effort" or "doing" approach. Little is mentioned about the "relaxed" or "non-doing" approach in sex, which is why we decided to write a book from the man's perspective. The non-doing approach is not a technique, but the opportunity to change yourself through changing the ways you express yourself sexually. The orientation is one of sexual union as a meditation in which the intelligence is handed back to the genitals.

Tantric Sex for Men also complements the previously published *Tantric Orgasm for Women*, which many men say is actually a book for men. Nonetheless, to explore sex specifically from the male perspective is of immense value. Readers are also referred to *The Heart of Tantric Sex: A Unique Guide to Love and Sexual Fulfillment*, which offers the "Love Keys" and many specific details about lovemaking that do not necessarily appear in this book. Here our intention is to offer a completely new picture of sex, one that brings about a revolutionary and evolutionary shift in the way we *think* about sex, and therefore express ourselves in sex. Through a change of mindset we can intentionally allow the body to relax into its inner wisdom and express itself as nature intended.

Our body of knowledge is based on personal experience and has been confirmed by thousands of couples who have passed through our weeklong residential "Making Love" retreats over the past twenty years. During the retreats there is no nudity, no partner swapping, and each couple arrives committed to each other for the week. The atmosphere is respectful, supportive, and professional. We sometimes share with couples how fortunate we feel to have the best work in the world. Actually, it is pure pleasure and not work at all. We experience unlimited joy in seeing couples rise in love out of stagnation right in front of our eyes, in a handful of days. This is not only one couple, but twenty-five or more couples simultaneously. Everything proceeds easily, gently, naturally, and with virtually no effort on our part.

Although sex has been practiced in certain ways for thousands of years, we don't believe it has to continue in the same way forever. Over the years we have come to recognize that changing the way we make love changes and empowers our lives in loving, magical, mystical ways. However, this kind of transformation happens only through direct experience, and not by simply thinking that it sounds like a great idea. To gain access to insider knowledge, the experience has to be lived fully by the individual on a cellular level. Transforming our basic sex energy into its higher vibration of love, as described in the chapters ahead, raises the quality of love on personal, social, and cosmic levels of consciousness.

During our time working in the field of sexuality some couples who have attended our retreats have naturally separated and gone different ways. Our approach is not foolproof; rather, it depends on individual awareness, curiosity, and an interest in change. To our great astonishment, over the years we have witnessed a steady trickle of men returning to our retreats with a new lover. Actions are said to speak louder than words, and the return of so many men is their living endorsement of the immense value of changing the way one makes love. Once a man has been fortunate enough to have a taste of his male potency flowing into and through a woman, and being received by her, he naturally hopes to create similar experiences for himself in the future.

Sometimes women are more ready than men to change their sexual ways. If your woman is ready to embark on an adventure into the unknown, follow her lead and let her take you to new horizons. Give it a whirl; there is really nothing to lose. Quite possibly you will gain more love and insight than you can imagine.

Humans have progressed in countless amazing ways, yet sex, the dimension closest to home, remains unexplored territory. Perhaps now is the time to move beyond the familiar and take a step in human sexual evolution.

To those men and women who have already taken this step and have written to us about their profound personal experiences, we extend our deep gratitude to you for allowing us to use your words in encouraging others to explore their sexual potential.

◈

Our spiritual master, Osho, formerly known as Bhagwan Shree Rajneesh, is the source of the tantric inspiration we now pass on to you. Osho's interpretation of the ancient Tantra scriptures addresses the search for harmony, wholeness, and love that is at the core of all religious and spiritual traditions, and that is also an integral aspect of the tantric relationship between two people. It is our privilege to include some excerpts of Osho's tantric inspiration throughout this book. His words, appearing in text form, were initially delivered as spontaneous oral discourses and later published in book form. The quotes included here are those that inspired us on our journey, and in no way represent the full range and extraordinary diversity of Osho's spiritual insight into the human condition.

We are both vitally aware that our lives have been shaped by Osho in ways that could not have been imagined at the outset, and for this honor we extend to him our eternal love and gratitude.

◈

Osho Speaks on Sex

Osho's Spiritual Insight into the Human Condition

I have almost four hundred books in my name. Out of four hundred books there is only one book on sex, and that too is not really on sex; it is basically on how to transcend sex, how to bring the energy of sex to a sublimated state, because it is our basic energy. It can produce life. . . . It is only man who has the privilege to change the character and the quality of sexual energy. The name of the book is *From Sex to Superconsciousness*—but nobody talks about superconsciousness. The book is about superconsciousness; sex is only to be the beginning, where everybody is.

There are methods that can start the energy moving upwards, and in the East, for at least ten thousand years, there has developed a special science, Tantra. There is no parallel in the West of such a science. For ten thousand years people have experimented with how sexual energy can become your spirituality, how your sexuality can become your spirituality. It is proved beyond doubt—thousands of people have gone through the transformation. Tantra seems to be the science that is, sooner or later, going to be accepted in the whole world, because people are suffering from all kinds of perversions. That's why they go on talking about sex as if that is my work, as if twenty-four hours a day I am talking about sex. Their repressed sexuality is the problem. My whole effort has been how to make your sex a natural, accepted phenomenon, so there is no repression—and then you don't need any pornography; so that there is no repression—and then you don't dream of sex. Then the energy can be transformed.

There are valid methods available through which the same energy that brings life to the world can bring a new life to you. That was the whole theme of the book. But nobody bothered about the theme, nobody bothered about why I have spoken on it. Just the word sex was in the title, and that was enough.

The book is not for sex; it is the only book in the whole existence against sex, but strange. . . . The book says that there is a way to go beyond sex, you can transcend sex—that's the meaning of "from sex to superconsciousness." You are at the stage of sex while you should be at the stage of superconsciousness. And the route is simple: sex just has to be part of your religious life, it has to be something sacred. Sex has to be something not obscene, not pornographic, not condemned, not repressed but immensely respected, because we are born out of it. It is our very life source. And to condemn the life source is to condemn everything. Sex has to be raised higher and higher to its ultimate peak. And that ultimate peak is *samadhi*, superconsciousness.

OSHO, TRANSCRIBED TEACHINGS,
SEX MATTERS: FROM SEX TO SUPERCONSCIOUSNESS

Tantric Inspiration

And about sex also people are very, very worried. That very worry and that very effort to do something is the problem. Sex happens; it is not a thing that you have to do. So you have to learn the eastern attitude toward sex, the Tantra attitude. The Tantra attitude is that you be loving to a person. There is no need to plan, there is no need to rehearse in the mind. There is no need to do anything in particular: just be loving and available. Go on playing with each other's energy. And when you start making love there is no need to make it great. Otherwise you will be pretending and so will the other person. He will pretend that he is a great lover and you will pretend that you are a great lover . . . and both are unsatisfied. There is no need to pose anything. It is a very silent prayer. Making love is meditation. It is sacred, it is the holiest of holies. So while you are making love, go very slowly . . . with taste, taking in every flavor of it. And very slowly: there is no hurry, no need to hurry, enough time is there.

OSHO, TRANSCRIBED TEACHINGS,
THE OPEN SECRET

1

MALE BURDEN OF PERFORMANCE

⬦━━━━⬦

Sex plays a central and crucial role in the life of a man from his early years onward, and remains significant regardless of whether a man is often having sex, seldom having sex, or not having sex at all. Since sex is pivotal to life, there are underlying aspects to the act that get hidden from sight, never brought into the light of day to be examined or questioned. Scratch the surface a little, however, and surprisingly soon men will start to express their feelings. Most men freely admit they would like to have sex more often, yet again and again they share with us in our seminars that as important as sex is, it is also experienced as a burden and a form of stress, which is sometimes subtle, other times not so subtle. The pressures implicit in sex can become a source of anxiety, which gives rise to a sense of insecurity and a lack of self-confidence.

When a man first gets together with a woman there is considerable pressure to be a good lover; perhaps he will even attempt to be the best lover this particular woman has ever had. There are many expectations, and the stakes are high. First, there has to be an erection, which is not guaranteed even in the most ideal situation, as we all know. Next, if and when the erection happens, it has to be maintained for as long as possible, which means that a certain level of stimulation and excitement is required. At the same time the man is praying that he doesn't ejaculate too quickly, at least not before the woman has her orgasm. And if everything works out just right, maybe it will even be possible to have an orgasm at the same time.

There are so many variables involved in the process that it is easy to get lost in the midst of monitoring and orchestrating the situation to best effect. At the beginning of a love affair a man's stress and performance anxiety are usually more obvious to him (but hopefully not to her), since he is more directly confronted by his wish to be successful. But after a while, as the relationship begins to unfold and assume a more day-to-day familiarity, his anxieties about performance temporarily bury themselves under a comfortable sexual routine. Even when a man is not consciously aware of his insecurity in sex, he nonetheless carries the emotional tension around with him each and every day of his life.

And in truth, the bottom line is that a woman can criticize a man about many things—being a lousy cook, a bad driver, unsuccessful at work, or even a miserable father. These criticisms are not easy to receive, but somehow they are manageable. But when a woman dares to criticize our sexual behavior, when she brings our performance into question, the words hit home and touch us at our most vulnerable place, rattling our male ego. To be not appreciated or valued as a lover can be very difficult for a man to digest.

RELAXING INSTEAD OF PERFORMING

Whether we are aware of it or not, much of our personality, identity, and self-perception is rooted in sex and in how we perceive ourselves as sexual beings. Sex also acts as a confirmation of our power and potency, thereby becoming connected—consciously or unconsciously—with pressure and performance in an attempt to prove our true value and worth.

Men who begin to experiment with a relaxed style of sex, as outlined in the chapters ahead, say it is an unbelievable relief to have the stress taken out of sex. All the big-time action that is unquestioningly accepted as part of sex simply falls away, because there is no longer a need for it. To relax in sex a man needs to be encouraged to abandon the idea that he, as the man, is 100 percent responsible for the quality of the shared sexual experience, whether it is very good, quite good, or unsatisfactory. In place of carrying the overall responsibility for the sexual interaction, which involves tremendous effort on his part, the man can discover how to simply *be* in sex—intensely present, in the here and now—and explore a more relaxing style of sex that does not include performance, effort, or tension.

Removing the Goal Removes the Pressure

In exploring a new style of sex, it is very helpful to shift our awareness from "doing" to "being." In order to alleviate performance pressure—the doing—the first step is to remove what we perceive as the goal. Generally the goal of sex is to have an orgasm. This goal of orgasm, which is the experience that usually makes people want to have sex in the first place, is what creates pressure. As we make love our deliberate intention and efforts are directed toward achieving that final end—a climax of heightened intense pleasure that lasts for a few short seconds.

There are significant disturbances that result from making orgasm the basic goal of sex. At the very outset, the focus on trying to get to the finish naturally causes us to get ahead of ourselves. This is true for men and women alike. If you pay attention you'll notice that your attention is more focused on the next penetration than the one happening right now in the present. Interest is generally in what lies ahead, what is coming next, and not what is occurring in the moment. The next penetration is more enticing because it brings us one step closer to the grand finale. We are unconsciously more focused on the future, so while the body remains engaged, there is little or no awareness of or in the present moment. We are following the mind with its specific ideas about how sex should go, and we are not tuning in and listening to the wisdom of the body.

Men often report wanting to have sex more frequently, but don't know how to make this happen. Many have lost confidence in reaching woman and have little clue as to how to get her more interested in sex. In our teaching we see how long-term issues like these begin dissolving in an extraordinarily short span of time—and only because of the non-goal-oriented, conscious style of sex we propose. During our retreats, we usually begin to see encouraging signs of response within individuals and between couples within two to five days. It is an honor to witness this miracle every time, like a shift from dark into light and from fear into love. All the barriers and problems that people arrived with begin to dissolve, and couples find a fresh sexual track leading to new dimensions, uncharted territory, and unlimited love. That it happens so easily is both astounding and reassuring.

Change Your Mind to Change Your Body

A shift of the kind experienced by our participants is possible *only* because the mind has reoriented to view sex and love from a diametrically opposite perspective. Without great effort you find you are indeed actually "making" love, and finally giving the expression its true meaning. When we stay present during lovemaking we naturally create love.

The solution appearing before us is quite simple—or so it seems! If we all change *our minds* about sex, we will possibly witness a dramatic reduction in the sex, love, and relationship problems to which people unhappily resign themselves.

HUMANS NEED MORE SEX

Sexual difficulties are experienced by both men and women, with the tragic outcome that human beings do not have enough sex. When sex finally happens the experience is short lived. Most partners do not have sex frequently enough for optimum mental, physical, and emotional health. Many do not make love for months and months on end, sometimes stretching into years. Sex satisfies our bodies, hearts, souls, intelligence, creativity, and most of all, our love—of self and of others. Sex is not the only way to access love, but if you are having or wanting sex, as most men are, then sex may as well be used to its highest potential.

When a U.K. satellite television channel recently conducted a survey on what people on their deathbeds regret most, seven out of ten British pensioners—both men and women—regretted not having "shagged around" (screwed around) more. As people were dying they were wishing they had had more sex in their lives. What an incredible revelation, that human beings are leaving this world sexually unfulfilled. Since it is becoming urgent and necessary for human beings to have more sex during their lifetimes, we need to develop a more evolved, sustainable style of sex that is manageable until our dying day. We need an approach that doesn't fizzle out when the newness is lost, disinterest or complacency sets in, or impotence or diminished hormones make sex more difficult.

EXPLORATION AND VULNERABILITY

To get more out of sex requires taking an adventurous step motivated by curiosity, intelligence, or both. The key is to make love frequently using the information and suggestions offered in the chapters ahead. If you follow where it leads and stay with what unfolds, you may soon notice a change in the quality of your life and a difference in how you feel about yourself as a man. You may even begin to perceive women differently.

As you begin to explore sex, old childhood wounds, memories, and insecurities may rise to the surface. It's better not to try to override or ignore any sexual difficulty or insecurity. Be open to yourself and allow your feelings to emerge, expressing any tears and vulnerability, not-knowing, insecurity, or confusion. Allowing yourself space to feel hidden aspects of your being is part of a healing and reintegrating process. Sexual exploration is a journey in self-discovery that not only leads to being a better lover with improved skills, but also can transform age-old restrictive patterns and generate more love and happiness. One thing is for certain—most women prefer a man's gentle, softer side to his hard, tougher side.

Rarely in the lifetime of the average human being are there altered states of orgasmic bliss, love, joy, and a peace that surpasses all understanding. The experience of being radiantly alive on a cellular level. Energized and aglow through merging with the body and its senses. Making love naturally presents us with an incredibly easy situation within which to "be present" and immerse ourselves in the body. Because of the absence of evolved sexual understanding, the human race suffers tremendous consequences. We are distorted by unconscious forces that affect our true nature, so that men are not truly men and women are not truly women. When we relate or connect through these distortions of our personalities and sexual identification, sooner or later the invariable result is tension and unhappiness.

SEXUAL CONDITIONING
AND HOW IT SHAPES US

Each of us is unconsciously conditioned by society whether we like it or not, some more heavily than others. In conventional sexuality the majority of men tend to demonstrate the distorted versions of their true male qualities. Below you'll find a list of true male qualities in the first column, each of which is followed by a word or a few words describing the same quality after it has been distorted through false sexual conditioning. The 1960s-era saying, "Make love, not war," is actually a truth. A lack of sufficient fulfilling or nourishing sex often results in anger and aggression. Changing a man's understanding, and therefore his experience of sex, naturally calls forth his original, authentic male qualities.

TRUE MALE QUALITIES VERSUS CONDITIONED DISTORTIONS

Power	Abuse, domination
Presence	Absence
Strength	Hardness
Clarity	Judgment
Assertiveness	Aggression
Creativity	Achievement, ambition
Meditation	Reclusiveness
Will	Stubbornness
Courage	Machismo, compensation
Leadership	Control, politics, law and order
Protector, authority	Authoritarian
Wildness	Brutality
Spontaneity	Performance
Wisdom	Arrogance
Charisma	Sexual manipulation
Sun, life giving	Sunburn, ecological destruction
Expression, articulation	Pomposity, boorishness
Action	Activity, bullishness
Independence	Isolation
Heartfelt, loving, compassionate	Selfish, egoistic

Tantric Inspiration

We live for sensations, we hanker for sensations. We go on seeking newer and newer sensations; our whole life is an effort to obtain new sensations. But what happens? The more you seek sensations, the less sensitive you become. Sensitivity is lost.

It looks paradoxical. In sensations, sensitivity is lost. Then you ask for more and more sensations and the "more" kills your sensitivity more. Then you ask for even more, and finally a moment comes when all your senses have become dull and dead. Man has never before been so dull and dead as he is today. He was always more alive before, because there were not so many possibilities to fulfill so many sensations. But now science, progress, civilization, education, have created so many opportunities to move further and further into the world of sensation. Ultimately, you turn into a dead person; your sensitivity is lost. Taste more foods—stronger tastes, stronger foods—and your taste will be lost. If you move around the world and go on seeing more and more beautiful things, you will become blind; the sensitivity of your eyes will be lost.

If you want the divine—the divine means the most alive, the ever-alive, ever-young, evergreen—if you want to meet the divine, you will have to be more alive. How to do it? Kill out all desire for sensation. Don't seek sensation, seek sensitivity, become more sensitive.

The two are different. If you ask for sensations you will ask for things; you will accumulate things. But if you ask for sensitivity, the whole work has to be done on your senses, not on things. You are not to accumulate things. You have to deepen your feelings, your heart, your eyes, your ears, your nose. Every sense should be deepened in such a way that it becomes capable of feeling the subtle.

OSHO, TRANSCRIBED TEACHINGS,
NEW ALCHEMY TO TURN YOU ON

2

INVOLUNTARY EJACULATION AND DESENSITIZATION

Perhaps the most common problem or issue faced by men is their lack of control over ejaculation, which results in an extremely high prevalence of premature ejaculation. And as we know, perhaps far too well, ejaculation usually marks the end of the sex act. As we come, we finish, at least for the present moment. Research has revealed that the universal average time of sexual engagement is between two and two-and-a-half minutes. Some men are able to extend the time to fifteen minutes, others to half an hour, or perhaps even forty-five minutes.

Enjoyable as these extra minutes definitely are, they are not really sufficient for a man to channel his vitality into a woman, and to have it received by her and returned to him. A man's ultimate fulfillment lies in being bathed in a woman's love, in overflowing radiant response to the love made in her. Man gives to woman who receives, and then woman gives to man who, in turn, receives. A reciprocal cycle of giving and receiving comes into play.

The truth is that if man wishes to make love for longer stretches of time and reap the true benefits of sex, then the level of excitement has to be drastically reduced and ejaculation consciously postponed.

EXCITEMENT CAUSES PREMATURE EJACULATION

Stimulation and excitement almost always end up in ejaculation. Yet at the same time it is a challenge to try to imagine sex without excitement. How would it look? What are you "doing" instead? Sex without excitement sounds like a contradiction in terms. Our impetus for wanting sex in the first place is precisely for sensation and intensity. After all, isn't that what sex is about?

Whether or not this is true for you, it is valuable to examine the role of excitement in conventional sex and perhaps come to the final conclusion that although excitement may be a great pleasure, too much of it can short-circuit the system. Facts are facts.

The basic problem doesn't lie with excitement per se, but rather with our sexual goals and the ways we manage the excitement. We begin sex with a strong intention, deliberately stimulate our bodies and genitals, and increase the level of intensity until there is a peak and overflow. These tactics basically produce too much heat, usually more than man can handle, so he boils over and discharges his life force, thereby unconsciously disempowering himself.

Sexual Fantasy Increases Excitement

Sexual fantasy is an accepted aspect of sex because it increases excitement. Fantasies in conventional sex are, in fact, a great help, but it is perhaps accurate to say that usually we are having sex with our minds, not with our bodies. We are unquestionably using our bodies, but we're not really understanding the way they are designed to function. Fantasy is a direct product of the mental powers of the imagination, and our bodies are forced to comply and satisfy the demands of our insatiable minds. As an example to show how sex and mind are connected, we remember a friend who told us that she had suffered an injury to her lower spine. This disturbance caused numbness and lack of sensitivity in the genitals over a period of several months. She couldn't feel a thing in her sexual organs. Nonetheless, she felt extreme desire for sex during this time. Finally she was forced to realize that the *source* of her sexuality lay in her mind, not in her body.

The mind is extremely powerful, but there are consequences to embracing fantasy as a sexual strategy. Fantasy is undeniably tied to excitement, which is tied to premature ejaculation; the three are linked together. Fantasy increases stimulation and excitement levels (as do all types of sexual aids), which in turn produce chronic premature ejaculation

Many people depend on fantasy and excitement for their sexual responses and in order to reach orgasm. The pornographic film industry is reportedly much larger than the mainstream film industry, and there are stripper bars in every major city in the world. Fantasy is an imagined situation; you are not with the person in the spirit of togetherness, sharing a mutual experience. You are mentally absent and not present, which results in the same consequence as focusing on the goal of orgasm; you are ahead of yourself or out of yourself. In both cases the mind, not the event itself, is the trigger. The mind wants orgasm and creates fantasy to satisfy its desire.

Staying Cool in Sex

If you want to avoid short-lived sex, it helps to heed an interesting folk aphorism: "A little is good, but more is not better." In the case of excitement this advice holds true; a little excitement is good, but more excitement is not better. Maybe more brings more pleasure and intensity, but if we wish to change, it's helpful to recognize the outcome of such behavior patterns.

In order to experience longer exchanges we need to cool down the sex act. A little excitement is fine, nothing is wrong in it, but then relax and take it easy. A retreat participant once shared his experience of having his thirty-year-old premature ejaculation problem vanish overnight, once he'd discovered the key of avoiding getting overexcited and remaining cool.

A style of sex that is cool and simple is more sustainable. It extends, expands, and increases the attraction between the bodies. The accepted cultural ideal is that sex should be as hot as possible, an approach that virtually guarantees premature ejaculation. Sooner or later excitement burns out, we take each other for granted, and boredom takes up residence. Boredom is natural; anything repeated again and again becomes a boring experience. Whenever the newness is lost, boredom takes its place. Excitement is triggered by the unknown, the newness of a situation, but the newness quickly wears off and the initial attraction burns up in the flames of excitement. Often couples report that after periods of heavy sex they experience a kind of physical repulsion and complete loss of interest in sex for a while.

SENSATION REDUCES SENSITIVITY

One significant by-product of excessive stimulation is that the penis becomes less and less sensitive. The more sensation to which the penis is subjected, the less sensitive it becomes. The same is true for the vagina. The repeated rubbing action of the penis within the vagina (or in the hand during masturbation) desensitizes both the penis and the vagina.

Repetitive in-and-out movements create friction between the tissues, which causes heat and a charge. After sex, a residue of tension remains in the body. This accumulates over time, and eventually the penis becomes subtly overcharged and tougher, and therefore less sensitive and less perceptive. Quite often the erect male penis feels unnaturally dense, hard, or even metallic to the touch. This rigidity reflects the tensions held in the tissue of the penis. Sensitivity is reduced, and a man loses the ability, capacity, and power to feel into the actual tissues of the penis. The penis itself loses inner vitality and consciousness, from its root all the way up to the radiant head. It forgets its slithering, supple, flexible nature that renders it capable of winding up and down inside the vagina exactly like a snake.

At the end of a retreat several years ago, a scientist who had participated told us that the loss of sensitivity in the face of intensity of stimulation had been scientifically proven in the second half of the nineteenth century by German physiologist Ernst Weber and physicist and psychologist Gustav Fechmer. Their research, formulated as the Weber-Fechmer law, is the theory of the relationship between stimulus and experience. Their research showed that the change in intensity of a sensation varies in increments proportional to the relative change of the stimulus. Today this is known to be true for every sensory channel within its range of dynamics. A simple example would be to light a match in the darkness. In this instance the light is like an explosion, but if you do the same in bright sunlight, it is barely perceptible. More sensation correlates to less sensitivity, and less sensation correlates to more sensitivity. Instead of endlessly seeking more and more sensation, we should begin to develop our senses so that we become capable of feeling the subtle yet vital life force moving through us at any moment of the day.

Mechanical Repetition and Loss of Sensitivity

To raise the intensity of sensation, we increase the tempo and frequency of our movements. We become mechanical, repeating the same thing again and again. Whenever there is an element of mechanical repetition in movement there is a corresponding lack of consciousness, and thereby loss of sensitivity, in each of the contributing individual movements. The steps that make up the journey are lost as we become climax machines, tense with the effort of getting where we want to go—orgasm!

Through being in a hurry we actually reduce the capacity to internally feel ourselves at a meaningful level. What is happening second by second in the body and genitals? Within the penis? Around the penis? Between the penis and vagina? If we are conscious in each moment, in each movement, the unfolding of sex can become a state of awe and wonder that lasts for hours. An experience of pure pleasure. A state of timelessness is entered wherein the moments emerge spontaneously from the body, unfolding naturally, one giving way to the next without fantasy or goals or mind being involved. The body is taken over by an innate force that intelligently guides it into loving expression. It is quite literally a mindless experience because we become utterly absorbed by our bodies in their state of heightened sesitivity. The more conscious and present a person is during sex, the greater his or her sensitivity will be.

Woman's Excitement Can Trigger Male Ejaculation

Most men have experienced coming very easily when the woman gets overexcited or too hot, especially as she strives to come to a climax. Ejaculation happens in a helpless enjoyable flash, and there is nothing to be done to avoid it. Many men confirm this experience, saying it is as if an ejaculation is virtually pulled from them, completely out of the blue. They are taken by surprise because they were nowhere near ready to ejaculate. Although the situation appears uncontrollable there is something that can be done, and that is to avoid making the woman too excited. If you'd like to make love last longer, maintain the sexual temperature at cool to gently simmering.

WOMEN'S SEXUAL RELUCTANCE

Let's face reality: men usually desire sex more often than their partners do. Ever wondered why? The truth is that for a woman the few minutes of sexual interaction are not really satisfying. There is hardly sufficient time for her body to warm up and celebrate the occasion. This sadly implies that women repeatedly return from sexual encounters feeling unfulfilled and at a loss—with the sense that the pleasures of sex are not worth the efforts of sex. Feelings such as these can get firmly embedded and cause many women to begin to avoid sex. Research reveals that 82 percent of women would rather kiss and cuddle than have sex; they find the exchange more nourishing. The choice to cuddle instead of having sex is a reflection of women's lack of true enjoyment when the penis is within the vagina.

Men can rest assured that the reluctant sexual response of a woman is not a mental or conscious response wherein she suddenly decides she does not want sex. (There are contraception issues that sometimes stand in the way of a woman's assent, mentioned in chapter 7.) The closing down of a woman's body is usually a slow, gradual process, unless she has suffered some trauma, in which case the closing down can be immediate. The withdrawal is physical yet very subtle, and something over which a woman does not have much conscious control. Many a woman feels she is alone in her unexpected and uninvited turnoff to sex, but it is a common and universal theme. Repeated lack of fulfillment plays a great part in why women experience loss of interest in sex. Women are definitely not frigid by nature, but their bodies start to freeze over when the sex is always hot, hard, and quick.

What's a man to do? Why precisely are women not enjoying sex? Why does your woman not want sex as much as you do? A recent *Redbook* survey shows that 52 percent of women regularly fake orgasms. According to a Durex Global Sex Survey, only 17 percent of women are likely to have an orgasm during sex. Forty-three percent of women report "some kind of sexual problem," such as the inability to achieve orgasm, boredom with sex, or total lack of interest in sex.

Basically women are not getting what they need sexually from men. At the root of the problems lies the male lack of understanding of the female body and man's loss of control over ejaculation. These facts are basic to female sexual withdrawal and difficulties in reaching orgasm. She doesn't enjoy sex because it doesn't feel good. How much sex would you want if you never even had an orgasm? If you want more sex from your woman, discover how to express yourself physically in a way that opens her, expands her body energy, and makes her ask for more. Once you figure that out, you won't have to ask. Trust us—she'll be asking you to make love to her. If you don't believe it, just try it.

There is an urgent need to discover how to extend the length of time of lovemaking, literally penis in vagina, for deeper sexual satisfaction of both the man and the woman. Their sexual experiences are inextricably intertwined, not separated into something one likes and the other does not. If a woman is not fully open to her partner, his sexual experience becomes one-dimensional, repetitive, and finally, boring. Then the need arises to introduce increasingly exciting and stimulating situations, porn movies, sex toys, party games, and the like to keep things rolling.

When woman is made love to consciously and at length, the man's experience is transformed; it becomes otherworldly, a multidimensional happening. When a man spends more clock time with his penis inside the woman he automatically thinks less about sex, because he is having it. Prolonged sexual experience in relaxation brings him a confidence and trust in himself, which in turn reduces presexual tension and excitement, and thereby postpones ejaculation.

Ejaculation can be postponed indefinitely once you discover the way to do so. Given that human beings do not make enough love, extending lovemaking by delaying, postponing, or even abandoning ejaculation sounds like the perfect remedy for bringing the situation into balance. There are always two opposing directions in which we can move with our sexual energy as human beings: emotional or mature, superficial or empowering, stimulating or relaxing, biological or spiritual, discharging or containing, reproductive or generative, unconscious or conscious.

PERSONAL SHARING
Enjoying Both Thrills and Silence

In the past six months of making love in silence without many outer movements, but with many more inner movements, it has become something that I had been seeking. It is the kind of making love that allows space for conscious encounters, deep love, unlimited variety, bubbling aliveness, powerful masculinity, and deep fulfillment. It is a wonderful path that leads me to who I truly am. At other times there is hot lovemaking with arousal. I experience excitement as something that pulls me in again and again. Sometimes it attracts me because I simply cannot let go of it, or it comes as a wave that overloads and overwhelms me. The experience is totally different from the silent lovemaking.

You taught us that, "Afterwards is your teacher." After the silent lovemaking I felt fulfilled and alive inside. After the love with excitement, in other words, after an orgasm, I felt tired and needed a break. In my personal experience there is another important difference. With the exciting love, I adhere to my partner energetically. In the silent love there is a space in which love can unfold between us. In regard to quality and sustainability, silent love is clearly leading for me, yet I'm not ready to say goodbye forever to lovemaking with excitement. I would be denying some parts in me that still long for that thrill, and I don't want to do that. I think further practice with tantra will lead the way. I allow myself to continue to be surprised as to where this path is taking me.

Tantric Inspiration

Ordinarily the energy is going outward and downward. You have to bring it backward, inward—and "inward" is synonymous with "upward." Once it starts coming back to you, and you become a circle of energy, you will be surprised: a new dimension has opened up; you start moving upward. Your life is no longer horizontal. It has taken a new route, the vertical.

OSHO, TRANSCRIBED TEACHINGS,
SECRET OF SECRETS

3

EJACULATION
IS NOT MALE ORGASM

The general assumption is that male ejaculation is a man's version of an orgasm. However, some men have discovered that ejaculation is definitely not a true orgasm. They have experienced that nature designed the genitals for elevated, or evolved, sexual experiences. They agree that ejaculation is an intense pleasure, but these few seconds cannot compare with the timeless, blissful, relaxing experience of orgasmic fusion. You find your body empowered, rejuvenated, and your spirits lifted.

Physiologically it is possible for man to have an orgasm without ejaculating. However, a man can also ejaculate sometimes without experiencing any pleasurable sensations whatsoever. Orgasm and ejaculation can occur simultaneously, or they can be experienced independent of one another. For a man this means he is capable of a prolonged "valley" orgasm, or even multiple orgasms, without ejaculation.

LOSS OF ENERGY AFTER EJACULATION

It is well known that men usually, or perhaps always, experience loss of energy after ejaculation. Signs of energy loss occur as a negative type of relaxation that is the result of the unburdening of accumulated tensions from the system. Stimulation and movement are used to build up tension levels; the breath gets shorter and faster until the energy peaks into a climax. Accumulated tension is discharged downward and outward along with life-giving semen (in contrast to the energizing effects of orgasm without ejaculation, which keeps the energy in the body and sends it vertically up the spine).

There are a number of ways in which the loss of energy after ejaculation manifests: a sense of separation, emptiness, loss of interest in the partner, irritability, tiredness, wanting to switch off, or falling asleep. There has been a depletion of energy, inducing a negative type of relaxation. The by-product of true relaxation is increased vitality and aliveness.

A young man of twenty-five years attended our weeklong seminar for couples, during which he immediately started to avoid ejaculation and contain his energy. After several days of making love two or three times a day without ejaculation, he observed a distinctly different quality arising from his body and his being, as though he had entered a love paradise. He felt as high as a kite.

Then, on the second to last afternoon he decided to have an ejaculation just to check it out and see how it would feel. He told us that from one second to the next he felt himself falling from heaven into hell. There was an instant evaporation of the positive, uplifting, inspiring inner force he had felt building up within himself during the previous days.

Since that shattering experience he has been able to observe and identify certain emotional and physical states that accompany or follow his ejaculation. Here is the list he made:

An intense idleness spreads inside of me.

Contact with people becomes difficult for me. I do not feel like seeing people.

The front of my torso is extremely tense for the next two days.

My lower back is contracted.

My neck is tense.

My body is generally tense. There is no space in me, no mobility.

I am irritable.

I behave like a child that did not get enough sleep, even if I've slept a lot.

Even little things are often too much. If I have to do something, it often feels like an insurmountable obstacle.

My thoughts are racing

I doubt my profession, my relationship, my living space, and my life. Nothing seems as good as it is.

I lack serenity. I feel no joy. I am afraid that everything will get to be too much.

My eyes are blurred and my head feels foggy.

I do not want to look at my beloved any more, and I am hardly able to look at her. If I do it anyway, I do not see her clearly.

I feel restless.

In brief, nothing is fun.

I need two to three days (at least) in order to recover, unless I start watching movies endlessly and avoid contact with anyone.

The rest of this man's interesting observations appear at the end of chapter 9.

The Power of Containment

The containment of sexual energy is not a new idea by any means. Containment was advocated and practiced by ancient Taoists and Tantrikas thousands of years ago and was considered pivotal to enjoying a long, healthy, creative, happy life.

Today, the majority of men (and women) never question ejaculation. With the equation ejaculation equals orgasm never being challenged, ejaculation becomes the goal of sex. It's why we do it. Besides, we think sex without a buildup and climax can hardly amount to real sex, and so ejaculation is given a central place without consideration of the many possible negative effects. Enormous amounts of spiritual and physical energy are required to rebalance and revitalize the system—energy that would otherwise be put to better use in essential body maintenance, especially as a man gets older.

One tablespoon of semen is unbelievably potent. The fluid contains an immense amount of proteins, vitamins, minerals, and amino acids, as well as vital energies. Semen is like liquid gold. With each ejaculation a man releases around forty million sperm cells, which have the potential to reproduce that many human beings. What incredible power!

Man unwittingly and habitually depletes his essence each time he has sex because of the prevailing idea that sex is for the pleasure of ejaculation.

The Spiritual Aspect of Sex Energy Rises

The creation of a human being is a miracle, yet the reproductive potential of sex is its more superficial expression. The higher, spiritual aspect of sex lies beyond the biological aspect, and this is where man differs fundamentally from his animal friends. Animal reproduction is relatively infrequent, generally limited to brief seasons, and occurs when the male of a species is attracted to specific odors emanating from the female. Sexual behavior is rarely displayed in the phases between seasons.

However, human beings are able to make love all day, every day if it is their individual wish, so there must be more to sex than straight-forward procreation. Man is able, through his consciousness, to raise his sexual expression to a higher level—one that is an evolutionary step. The containment of the life force through relaxation gives rise to still-ness and a higher form of self-experience. Sexual experiences become uplifting, deeply moving, and nourishing. Further, the capacity to be relaxed in sex and avoid tension-filled climax-oriented sex gives rise to a quality of male authority and presence that is lacking today in the majority of men. (This aspect will be covered in chapter 8.)

A man's experience of the spiritual aspects of sex is limited because there is confusion about sex. Nature has an inherent commitment to reproduction (among all plant and animal species) and is not at all interested in states of ecstasy or fulfillment of orgasmic potential. Ejaculation, which serves nature perfectly well, also leads to a crash landing well before humans take off and start flying. The usual brevity of the sex act means that the majority of men are not experiencing the vagina as the true home and resting place of both man and penis. In a man's lifetime inestimable amounts of time and energy are locked up into sexual fantasy and longing, but the actual amount of time a man spends with his penis inside a vagina is minimal.

A style of superficial reproductive sex is basically not satisfying in the long term. Again and again the longing to repeat the same experi-ence arises and can become a vicious cycle of desire and discharge. With repetition boredom easily sets in, so a man will change partners in order to keep his sex life alive.

When the ejaculation experience is truly fulfilling there is a sense of deep satisfaction and completion. Instead, most men, as already mentioned, feel depleted and devoid of creativity. Because the peak climax is not profound or deeply touching, the desire for sex continues almost as a compulsion or an obsession, and a man can find himself fully controlled by his sexual urges.

With the habit of building up and discharging energy the more subtle, delicate layer of sexual experience is bypassed. The life force is not given the opportunity to circulate within the body. Ejaculation interrupts the circle, and the higher potential of sex is lost. When a man learns to experience his higher orgasmic nature and finds deeper fulfillment through sex, there usually will be a corresponding decrease in his sexual obsession.

CONTAINING THE LIFE FORCE

For a man to shift gears and reach a higher octave in sex, he needs to prolong the sex act by cooling down and either avoiding ejaculation or postponing it until a moment of his choosing. The bodies of a man and a woman need to make love for an extended period of time for states of sexual ecstasy to arise. The human body is designed by nature to experience higher states, but this requires time, sensitivity, and awareness.

If a man understands that premature ejaculation happens through overexcitement, he can make ejaculation a conscious choice, rather than an accident or a habit, as mentioned in the previous chapter. Tantra masters also inform us that ejaculation is always preceded by the thought of ejaculation, that the origin of ejaculation is actually in the mind. Without the thought of ejaculation there is rarely an ejaculation (except when a woman gets overexcited and pulls an ejaculation from a man, as already mentioned).

Avoid the Tension of Ejaculation Control

Absence of ejaculation (nonejaculation) is not the same as ejaculation control. There is a significant difference between not ejaculating as a result of relaxation and controlling the ejaculation.

Osho says, "In sex, you are relaxing in it, not controlling it. If you are controlling it, there will be no relaxation. If you are controlling it, sooner or later you will be hurried to finish it because control is a strain. And every strain creates tension, and tension creates a necessity, a need, to release. It is not control; you are not resisting something. You are simply not in a hurry because sex is not happening in order to move somewhere. You are not going somewhere. It is just a play; there is no goal. Nothing is to be reached, so why hurry?"

This is different from sexual practices that suggest a man "dance on the verge" of ejaculation for a period of time without actually ever getting to the point of ejaculation. In other words, the man intentionally builds up the excitement and tension level, and then shortly before he feels he is about to reach the "point of no return," he relaxes his efforts, which represses the ejaculation. After a while the energy level is built up again, and then repressed again, and this process is continued with the effect that ejaculation is controlled for a prolonged period. (There are also specific techniques to repress ejaculation; for example, a man pushes finger pressure into his perineum/prostate area.) As the term *controlling ejaculation* indicates, by using such repressive techniques, the shift is from ejaculation to avoiding ejaculation—which means that the goal orientation remains the same.

Physical Pain after Hot Sex

Controlling ejaculation through repression as described above can have a short-term energizing effect on a man. However, the deliberate building up and pushing down of excitement will deposit tension in the prostate gland and genitals, which can later cause congestion. Because all repression is basically a type of tension, the practice of ejaculation control is not particularly healthy in the long term. When a man deliberately plays with excitement and controls his ejaculation, he should not be surprised if he experiences pain in the testicles or groin area afterward. The pain is usually a reflection of the tension produced through the buildup and repression of energy.

If, and when, a man does reach a point where he needs to ejaculate, it's suggested that he simply allow it to happen right then and there. Better not to interfere with the direction of the flow. Tell your woman out loud in words that you are coming, look into her eyes, remain present to the situation, and enjoy!

If you wish to postpone or avoid ejaculation, it's advisable to steer clear of too much stimulation and excitement right from the start of the lovemaking. Instead, become more slow and sensitive through relaxation and awareness. A cool approach can empower you to make love for hours.

Pain that Follows Relaxed Sex

After relaxed sex, surprisingly enough, there can also be pain in the penis, the testicles, the groin area, or the lower abdomen. When the sexual atmosphere has been one of relaxation, the pains are informing us that previously held accumulated tensions are leaving the tissues. These can be called "healing pains." If this should happen to you, accept the pain and do not be unduly concerned; the pain will pass in time. Movements such as gently shaking the body, including the pelvis, for ten minutes or more will help to disperse the emerging tensions. Often allowing simple tears of vulnerability will dissolve the pain. It is also recommended that masturbation not be used as a way to relieve the tension or pain. The body is healing and regenerating itself through the sexual relaxation. As layers of emotion and physical tensions rise to the surface and dissolve, body sensitivity and capacity for pleasure return.

Safety Concerns Regarding Nonejaculation

We have heard from a few men that they have been advised by their medical doctors to ejaculate regularly in order to "flush out the pipes," like a bit of do-it-yourself plumbing.

Personal experience has proved that it is possible to make love frequently for years on end without the need for ejaculation. It is not as though a man swells up into a balloon that eventually pops because of his unreleased semen! There is absolutely no physical danger for a man to go without ejaculation indefinitely. Sometimes there may be spontaneous emissions during the night, but these tend to happen more and more rarely as time passes. They occur frequently during puberty and adolescence, and the reason is thought to be sexual fantasies. These emissions have nothing to do with not having had an ejaculation for a long time or the body getting rid of old sperm.

Reserve Ejaculation for Conception

A man can, if he so wishes, reserve his ejaculation for procreation alone. There is no hard-and-fast rule, but a man should know that when he and his partner want to conceive, he can consciously decide to ejaculate at the time the woman is ovulating. (The time of ovulation can be determined through a number of different methods, such as changes in body temperature and vaginal mucus.) Conscious ejaculation will make conception an equally conscious event, rather than the hit-or-miss accident it often is. When a man ejaculates he can plant his seed along with an intention or vision for a conscious conception.

Women's Identification with Male Ejaculation

Men need to be aware that women often identify with their man's orgasm/ejaculation. In these few moments a woman feels that the man gives himself to her, and for woman this is somehow affirming. The irony is that she actually triggers the man into postejaculation syndromes, unwittingly disempowering him (and thereby herself) as the flow of intimacy and love gets interrupted or evaporates. Sometimes these breaks in the connection seem so normal that we would not immediately associate them with sex. We think this is who we are and how we are. However, a man who practices containment of energy will begin to experience himself as a completely different person in his daily life. Men report feelings of pleasure that rise to the heart with a lightness and glowing warmth that radiates throughout the entire body and being.

A man is equally identified with the woman's orgasm, because it confirms that he is a good lover, which supports the male ego. (However, many woman fake orgasm, so it is not necessarily reliable feedback.) The big disadvantage of making a woman come, as mentioned earlier, is that more often than not the man will ejaculate a few seconds too early due to the heightened level of excitement and tension, and so disempower himself.

BENEFITS OF COOLING DOWN

Many of the personality difficulties or relationship problems between partners disappear when there is a shift in the style of sex. An ambience of love surrounds the lovers, and radiant love shines from their eyes. Men's faces change completely when they are making love regularly in a relaxed, non-orgasm-focused way. The transformation is remarkable, certainly more effective than any facelift. Craggy, angular, mildly discontented grooves and folds transform into a widening and fullness of the face, as an infusion of *chi* or *prana,* the life force, enters into the facial tissues, energizing and rejuvenating the skin and leaving it rosy and radiant. The body is grounded as legs penetrate the earth; the heart is open, the eyes are shining.

Redirecting the Energy

In conventional sex the energy or vitality is normally forced downward and outward. To reach orgasmic states the energy has to be allowed to rise. It needs to be encouraged inward and upward, and this happens through relaxation in sex. An inner channel opens, and energy begins rising and expanding through the core, returning to its source in the brain. The ultimate source of the sexual energy lies in the brain. Roughly at the level of third eye lie the pineal and pituitary glands, known as the "master glands" of the endocrine (hormonal) system. Crucial substances and information are released and these filter downward through the system to eventually prepare us for sex. This cycle represents the reproductive, biological phase of sex mentioned earlier. When vitality is recirculated upward through inner channels and returns to its source in the brain it represents the spiritual or generative phase of sex. The inner design enables a man to reabsorb his vital energies and be empowered by them. Through relaxation a man can reach a vibrant and peaceful state, followed by the experience of feeling energized and rejuvenated.

It is an experience beyond and higher than the conventional reproductive expression, which is more "superficial." By allowing the life force to turn inward and upward, the man uses his intention to create the foundation for evolved experiences. He shifts from running mechanically after ejaculation to being conscious and present each moment, attentive to the subtle sensations unfolding within his body and being.

The Inner Rod of Magnetism

Perhaps you are wondering how these altered states transpire. What's going on? Both the male and female orgasmic experience can be explained most simply by comparing the human body to a magnet. Like a magnet, the body has two opposite poles—one in the heart and one in the genitals. Usually one pole is given a plus, or positive value, and the other a minus, or negative value. Whatever symbol or words you choose to use, the body's two equal and opposite poles create a difference in potential. This can give rise to an electromagnetic streaming in the core of the body and an amplification of the energy field surrounding the body. Tantra calls the experience of streaming in the core the awakening of the "inner rod of magnetism." And this is the true source of the human being's orgasmic experience. Through this miraculous inner design humans are able to experience ecstasy, alone or together.

Recent studies of chromosomes confirm the "magnetic" design of human beings. Science has proven that man is part woman, and woman is part man. Each human contains both parts, male and female. Both opposing poles are contained within each individual. We each have a male and a female pole, a heart pole and a genital pole. Each individual is, at a higher level and by design, an independent unit unto himself. Each person has the innate capacity to circulate energy and vitality within his or her self, which is ultimately the experience of "inner sex" and the most evolved form of human sexual expression.

PERSONAL SHARING
My First Full-Body Orgasm

I'm in India and it is 1993. I have been here more than a month, meditating every day, and suddenly I fall in love. It happens instantly, just by looking at her. We meet the first day of a meditative therapy that lasts three weeks, and after a couple of weeks of courting and wooing we meet at her home to make love. After long foreplay we get into the real act. Since I arrived in India I have not had any sexual contact with a woman, so even though I'm in ecstasy about making love with the woman I most desire in the whole world, I also have the classic male fear—some call it performance anxiety—that makes me think, "I hope I don't come immediately."

For me the first love encounter with a woman has always been like a testing ground: If the feeling is real, everything goes well and the experience is satisfactory for both partners; if it is not a real energetic feeling but the mind comes between us, then the experience is not satisfactory. On this night all best conditions are met—there is heart, our bodies like each other, and very importantly, we are both meditating regularly. I have always been a sensitive man, but tonight is pure magic. I can feel what she feels and I know exactly where, and how, and when to touch her. I really feel like I am one with her. The embrace really lasts a long time and every anxious thought is completely gone and I am totally relaxed.

The moment comes when she reaches orgasm and I, too, am captured by the escalation of pleasure that usually leads to a short, intense little squirt that we usually call "male orgasm." But this time it's different. In the beginning everything goes as usual, with the energy concentrating in my penis, ready to be scattered outside. This time, however, instead of going out, the energy goes up my entire body, shaking me in powerful waves. It could be described as a tremor, because the body can't be still, and there is heat, a kind of inner tingling, waves of pleasure everywhere, and maybe women can relate to this . . . these waves are not focused on the penis but wash through my whole body, all the way to my crown. Initially the interval between these long pleasure waves is a few seconds, and then they become less frequent, with longer intervals.

I feel the energy rushing through my body, flowing from me to her, *going through her body and coming back to mine through the contact between penis and vagina. I realize that if we keep a light contact with our tongues the waves pass more easily from my body to hers, creating a virtual circle that lasts long and eventually fades slowly, slowly . . . and it is beautiful to lie together, hugging, to watch the shaking of our bodies, the energy waves going up and down the spine, exchanging that state of ecstasy, indefinitely recharging each other. And when the waves calm and my ocean becomes still again I have the usual post-orgasm symptoms: my penis becomes soft again and my limbs are relaxed.*

Since that first time it has happened many times, but not always. This kind of orgasm, the valley orgasm, just happens of its own accord; I can't make it happen, I can only relax and allow it to happen. The biggest difference from a traditional orgasm is that after making love it takes less time for me to be ready again, because I've gained energy rather than wasting it, and the feeling of desire is untouched. After a night of these orgasms I need less sleep than usual, only a couple of hours, to be okay and get up perfectly refreshed. If I don't ejaculate I can go on making love for hours and hours. Of course I don't mean the boring "in and out" that we usually mean by making love. I mean following the energy, allowing the energy to guide me to move, to slow down, to stop . . . I wait, feeling what happens in my and her body, feeling the exchange of energy that goes through my penis.

The most important thing for me is to be relaxed. When I feel pleasure rising intensely, I have to remember to relax, rather than becoming tense as I normally would. It is particularly important to keep the muscles of the anus relaxed and soft, not tight and contracted. This expansion allows energy to go free, rather than being obstructed there: if the energy can't find the space to go up, it will be forced to go down into an ejaculation.

The other important thing is meditation. I've noticed that this type of orgasm is more likely to happen when I'm meditating regularly.

I don't think that technical knowledge about tantra is particularly important. That first time, in 1993, I was so completely ignorant about tantra that I was surprised and puzzled about what was happening to me, and thought I might be ill. I had to wait for years, till I met you both in 2000, to learn more about the circulation of energy in and between male and female bodies.

Tantric Inspiration

Tantra says do not try to escape; there is no escape possible. Rather, use nature itself to transcend. Don't fight—accept nature in order to transcend it. If this communion with your beloved or your lover is prolonged with no end in mind, then you can just remain in the beginning. Excitement is energy. You can lose it; you can come to a peak. Then the energy is lost and a depression will follow, a weakness will follow. You take it as relaxation, but it is negative.

Tantra gives you a dimension of higher relaxation, which is positive. Both partners melting with each other give vital energy to each other. They become a circle, and their energy begins to move in a circle. They are giving life to each other, renewing life. No energy is lost. Rather, more energy is gained because through the contact with the opposite sex your every cell is challenged, excited.

And if you can merge into that excitement without leading it to a peak, if you can remain in the beginning without becoming hot, just remaining warm, then those two warmths will meet and you can prolong the act for a very long time. With no ejaculation, with no throwing energy out, it becomes a meditation, and through it you become whole. Through it your split personality is no more split: it is bridged.

OSHO, TRANSCRIBED TEACHINGS,
VIGYAN BHAIRAV TANTRA

4

THE EQUAL AND OPPOSITE FORCE OF THE FEMALE ENVIRONMENT

◆━━━━━━◆

MEN AND WOMEN
ARE NOT THE SAME

Much of the confusion and misunderstanding that occurs between men and women results from ignorance regarding our true differences. These deep-seated differences shape our respective roles during sexual communion. With insight into these differences we can begin to work together to reveal and unleash our sexual potential.

For deeper insight into our human potential we refer to information contained in the Tantras (the tantric scriptures), sacred knowledge from the ancients. These ancient sources contain compelling information that rightfully should be passed down from one generation to the next.

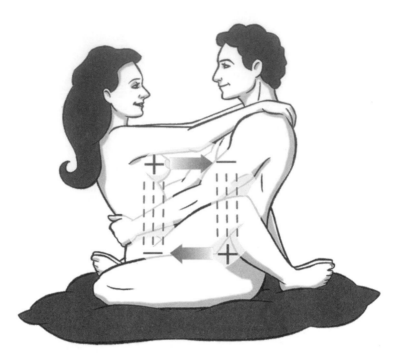

Fig. 4.1. Inner magnets of man and woman, showing poles, magnetic rods, and potential circular energy flow (in yab-yum position).

Male and Female Aspects within the Individual

The previous chapter explained the way in which each human being can be likened to a magnet, with a male and a female pole energetically linked by a rod of magnetism that, when awakened, gives rise to an inner electromagnetic streaming. This subtle internal by-product of the inner male and female forces at play within us represents our innate bisexual reality, and represents the very foundation of tantra and the biological basis of the orgasmic experience.

Of particular significance is that these two forces are equal. One is not more, one is not less; they are balanced, even. However, these poles simultaneously exist as opposite forces in relation to each other. The poles are equal forces, but opposite forces, not identical forces. Male represents an outgoing—"positive" or dynamic—force. Female represents a receptive—"negative" or passive—force.

The qualities of receptive and dynamic are diametrically opposite, and at the same time, they are equal and opposite and complement each other. They balance, correspond, and enhance each other, and one cannot exist without the other. Just as electricity requires two poles, positive and negative, no being or body can be without two poles, masculine and feminine, the universal forces of yin and yang.

Dynamic and Receptive Poles

In the male body the male, positive pole is represented in the genitals, the female, receptive pole in the chest/heart. The reverse is true for woman; the male, positive pole is in the breasts/nipples/heart, the female, receptive pole is in the genitals. When man and woman are in an upright, standing position, man can be visualized as a magnet standing on its head, with the positive (north) pole below and the negative (south) pole above. The woman is like a magnet standing upright: the positive (north) pole is above and the negative (south) pole is below.

Magnets Meet at Opposite Ends

When a man and a woman come together in an embrace, for instance, their bodies actually meet with energetically opposite ends aligned. The positives and negatives of each individual approach and meet simultaneously at the genital and heart levels. The inner rods of magnetism (as mentioned in the previous chapter as the source of the orgasmic state) flow in opposite directions to each other. When two magnets meet at opposite ends, there is an attractive force that pulls them together. And the same "magnetic" attraction can also be felt between male and female bodies. There is a perceptible drawing and pulling sensation as the equal and opposite forces influence each other. In addition, there is tremendous amplification of the magnetic or energy fields surrounding the two magnets/bodies.

The Dynamic Male Force

A man's body contains two poles, but the male dynamic aspect is the outer aspect, while the female (receptive) is his inner aspect. In a woman's body the reverse is true. The female receptive aspect is outer, and the male (dynamic) aspect is her inner aspect. One aspect is externalized, but both aspects are always present. Generally speaking, this implies that physically and energetically the man, predominantly male, is a dynamic force, while the woman, predominantly female, is a receptive force. Man does not have to take any direct action to connect with his feminine side, or his so-called inner woman. The more truly male man becomes through a relaxed, non-doing presence in sex, the more his opposite feminine quality of love will naturally and gradually open up. There will be a balancing within him. Similarly, a woman will access her "inner man" by relaxing increasingly into her feminine nature. The harmonizing inner opposite emerges and flowers as an alchemical process, as an outcome or a by-product.

Figure 4.1 shows the inner magnets of a man and woman with poles, magnetic rod, and potential circular energy flow while sitting in yab-yum position.

Genitals—Equal and Opposite Forces

The qualities of these forces, the intrinsically different polarities of man and woman, extend down to the level of the genital tissues. The shape of the male penis informs us that it is an instrument from which energy can flow or emanate. Likewise, the vagina is shaped as a canal or receptor with an innate capacity to receive, absorb, or draw out the opposite force.

Energetically and physically our equal and opposite forces are complementary; they fit together to form a single unit. There is a completion in the joining of the penis and vagina, when a man's dynamic pole meets and penetrates a woman's receptive pole. When separate and apart, it can be said that the genitals exist as two incomplete halves. Tantra masters believe that everything that is incomplete is longing for completion and suggest that the search for sex, the longing for sex, represents a deep yearning for union, completion, and peace.

Through the understanding of polarity—the equal, opposite, and complementary forces—it becomes more apparent that man is not necessarily an independent unit unto himself. In order to invite the truly masculine qualities embodied in his penis, a man is dependent on the environment around him, namely, the vagina. The quality of receptivity determines or influences the dynamic qualities. A dynamic force can only be dynamic (experience its very self) through being received. In fact, the more receptive, the more dynamic; the two happenings are inextricably linked. Giving makes receiving possible, and receiving makes giving possible, which is why it is so important for a man to take into account his equal and opposite force and become aware of the vital role of receptivity.

The Significance of the Female Environment

To manifest the vitality of the penis and discover how best to call forth its dynamic male qualities (and essential function), the woman needs to be centrally placed in the sexual constellation. Man physically enters woman with his penis, so the environment surrounding the penis is to be given value and not underestimated. The polarity differences between men and women are best embraced and enhanced, not sidestepped, in order to make the most of the sexual situation. Acknowledging the woman's receptive nature allows the man to experience himself as a truly masculine force. He feels a deep sexual fulfillment when he experiences male energy flowing through him and being received by the woman.

Man is inextricably dependant on woman for his higher experiences, and her environment needs some preparation to be able to warmly receive the guest. Man basically can be ready for sex at any given moment if he so wishes, which is probably the by-product of being a positive, dynamic force. Woman's lack of instant readiness is a by-product of her nature as a receptive, passive force. Any reluctance or unwillingness in sex is not a mental hang-up or frigidity, but rather a reflection of the intelligence of the body.

Woman's Body Needs Clock Time to Open

Usually man prefers to penetrate woman as soon as possible. Getting inside her becomes his primary focus, often from fear of losing his initial erection response. When a man has to hang around on the fringes waiting for the woman, he easily loses his erection and may have to wait some time for another. In reality, a leisurely, extended time frame, even an hour or three, will normally suit woman very nicely. She is able to tune into her body and relax into herself. If the man takes the time to "be" with the woman, perhaps to lovingly and softly (as a feather) caress her body into an energetically expanded state *before* entering her, he will be amazed by what an awesome experience it is. To consciously enter and be received by an inviting and absorbing channel changes the entire experience, which in turn transforms man.

When woman is entered too early, without feeling truly ready to receive, without the feeling of a total yearning "yes," her body may begin gradually to close down, interest in sex may dwindle, and reluctance to have sex may increase. During the initial phases of lovers' meeting, the woman's heart is wide open, so receiving man totally and at any time is not an issue. But sooner or later a woman will require acknowledgment of her differences if she is to continue enjoying sex well into her later years. The same is true for man. On an encouraging note, once a man of eighty years attended a couple's workshop with his wife of seventy-six; four years later they continue to have genital union as a daily practice. Their motivation in attending was to have one more adventure in life, and they both report a vastly improved quality of life; each day is a joy and filled with love.

When man enters a woman before her body is "open," it is similar to butting his head against a closed door. You can get only so far, but no further. However, when you have the keys to the door, you will find it opens easily and often. When man accepts the fact that woman is basically slower than he and her system requires preparation, then his sexual experiences will begin to transform into empowering acts of love.

Energy flows from positive to negative. This is the direction of movement, penis into vagina. A doorway opens, energy moves. When woman is vibrantly receptive, the direct connection between penis and vagina forms one vital unit. There is a flow and exchange of energy, potency, and life force.

The Diminished Role of the Clitoris in Tantric Sex

The vagina naturally has greater significance (for both men and women) than the clitoris because it is understood to be the receptacle for man's dynamic force. Normally the clitoris is considered to be the saving grace, the sun around which everything revolves, because clitoral stimulation can easily, but not necessarily, bring woman to orgasm. Clitoral stimulation will intensify excitement, which can, in fact, have a subtly disturbing effect on the cellular receptivity of the vagina. This tension in turn disturbs the capacity of woman to accept and receive the dynamic force into her. Clitoral stimulation elicits sexual desire but causes tension and confusion in the vaginal vibration, and the potential of the penetration is reduced.

Basic to experiencing higher states is maintaining a lower level of excitement, as introduced in chapter 2. A cool, nonstimulating approach allows the vagina to remain free of tension, able to maintain a relaxed, receptive atmosphere. If a woman is able to monitor her own excitement, to relax into her body rather than work at building up the intensity, she is less likely to inadvertently trigger man's ejaculation. Likewise, if man does not attempt to excite his woman, ejaculation can be postponed and lovemaking can be extended for hours.

A woman can get a bit fixated on her clitoris because of the pleasure and intensity experienced though these nerve endings. Sometimes it can be challenging to let go of things we know and have enjoyed. All the same, an elevation of sexual experience requires curiosity and intelligence by both partners and a willingness to explore the unknown. (See chapter 8 for more about the clitoris.)

Female Sexual Energy Is Raised in the Breasts

The big question is now how to knock on heaven's door. The true way to expand female sexual energy is to initially shift the emphasis away from the vagina and clitoris toward the breasts, which signifies *a shift from negative pole to positive pole in woman.* The breasts are the positive, dynamic pole from which energy is awakened, the key to accessing the female body. Energy can only be raised from a positive, dynamic pole and not from a passive, receptive pole. First the breasts need to become energized and filled with awareness (and this takes time), and then as a result the vagina will respond and become an invitation. Through merging with her breasts a woman is capable of experiencing the most profound orgasmic states. The vagina/clitoris, which is the usual starting point in conventional sex, is—energetically speaking—the passive, receptive pole in the female body. In truth, the vagina can only become fully alive and energized via the positive and dynamic pole of the breasts.

When man knows that the breasts are the doorway, the access to woman, his approach can be simpler and more informed, with less guessing or fiddling around to find the clitoris and get it just right. Instead, loving attention can be given to the breasts, which doesn't even require much effort on man's part. It is more a matter of "being" in your hands, without any intention or agenda lying behind the touch. A warm hand that gently embraces and lovingly molds to the breasts is absolutely perfect. There is no need to stimulate the nipples directly, but only indirectly through simple hand contact or a feather-light brush once or twice. Some women have hypersensitive nipples, so it's best to find out what suits your woman. (See more on breasts and foreplay in chapter 7.)

Ancient tantric wisdom makes it possible to initiate a thrilling journey of self-discovery, the outcome of which is the true experience of masculinity. This requires a revolutionary reevaluation of sex and the discovery that the "how" of sex plays a profound role in maintaining an active sex life and a loving, joyful relationship. The key is to treat woman as complementary and not the same. Any limitation in the sexual experience of woman inevitably limits the sexual experience of man. If woman is adversely affected through a lack of orgasmic experiences, then so is man, even if he is not aware of this.

SHIFT FROM SENSATION TO SENSITIVITY

There is a general requirement to shift away from sensation and excitement toward sensitivity and nature's subtle energetic connection.

Lovemaking must be reconceived as an interplay of dynamic and receptive forces that give rise to extraordinary energetic experiences. A shift away from sensation toward sensitivity imbues man with true male attributes and the ability to be present to his penis. To give value to, and opportunity for, the male-female connection within the vagina, where the vagina becomes an embracing sheath that elicits the essential qualities imbued in the penis, supporting man's experience of himself as authentic man. A natural biological ecstasy is possible, an exchange that satisfies every cell in the body and lies beyond the pleasure of ejaculation and fantasy.

The penis has a definite intelligence and innate sensitivity. When the female environment is open, warm, and loving, the penis responds positively to the intrinsic force-flow. When the female environment is closed, tight, or unwelcoming, the penis can easily shrink and withdraw as it loses cellular interest. For a man it is a profoundly moving and touching experience to feel deeply welcomed into the vagina by a woman.

Awakening Polarity

You and your partner can make yourselves more aware of your complementary polarities before you start lovemaking—as a kind of foreplay. Or at any other time.

Sit opposite each other on the floor on cushions situated a little distance apart so that your knees or hands aren't touching. Close your eyes and tune into your positive poles: for you that would be at the root of your penis (the perineum), and for your partner, her breasts and nipples. Take a few minutes for this. After a while when you feel you have managed to pull your attention into your penis and testicles, imagine the penis radiating energy, light, and warmth toward your woman's vagina. She should imagine herself receiving the love and light into her vagina and at the same time radiating warmth, light, and love out through her breasts to you. Imagine receiving all this beautiful energy and absorb it into your chest and heart.

You can use the breath to support the experience if you wish (but should you feel more relaxed without any special attention on the breath, this choice is fine too). As you breathe out, radiate love and light from the penis. As you breathe in, absorb the love and light coming from her breasts. Breathe in together and then out together for a while. Or as one breathes out, the other breathes in, then vice versa. When you feel ready, open your eyes in a gentle, receptive way, and sustain an inviting, gentle eye contact.

If you feel a physical attraction arising between you, woman can move across the space, and you can assist her to wrap her legs around your waist while sitting in your lap (yab yum position); cushions can be used to support her if necessary. This position brings the genitals into closer proximity and the breasts and chest into correspondence. This means the inner magnets are meeting at opposite ends. Embrace lightly and feel the inner sensations, or use the imagination to circle the energies.

If you wish, you can also change the breathing pattern—as you breathe in, woman breathes out; as woman breathes in, you breathe out. This practice will intensify the feeling of the energy and aliveness circling between your bodies. After a time you probably will begin to feel subtle sensations of the energy circulating. If yab-yum is not comfortable to sustain, you can move into a standing position, or you can do the entire exercise standing. Experiencing this circling energy may lead to a mutual desire for union, but if not, slowly separate your bodies so that you don't suddenly break the energetic connection. Sit with closed eyes and settle your attention inside your own body for few minutes.

Tantric Inspiration

And this merger should not become unconscious, otherwise you miss the point. Then it is a beautiful sex act, but not transformation. It is beautiful, nothing is wrong in it, but it is not transformation. And if it is unconscious then you will always be moving in a rut. Again and again you will want to have this experience. The experience is beautiful as far as it goes, but it will become a routine. And each time you have it, again more desire is created. The more you have it, the more you desire it, and you move in a vicious circle. You don't grow, you just rotate.

Rotation is bad because then growth is not happening. The energy is simply wasted. Even if the experience is good, the energy is wasted, because much more was possible. And it was just at the corner, just a turn, and much more was possible. With the same energy the divine could have been achieved. With the same energy the ultimate ecstasy is possible, and you are wasting that energy in momentary experiences. And by and by those experiences will become boring, because repeated again and again, everything becomes boring. When the newness is lost, boredom is created.

If you remain alert you will see: first, changes of energy in the body; second, dropping of thoughts from the mind; and third, dropping of the ego from the heart. And when this third thing has happened, that energy, your sex energy, has transformed into meditative energy.

OSHO, TRANSCRIBED TEACHINGS,
MY WAY: THE WAY OF THE WHITE CLOUDS

5

THE PENIS—A POTENT ELECTROMAGNETIC INSTRUMENT

A man who experiences his penis as a divine instrument of love and ecstasy develops a profound trust in his manhood, which rests easily and gently at the center of his being. He has the capacity to listen to his body, loves and respects his penis, and knows how to be male in relation to female. He understands the source of his erection and is in control of his ejaculation, and not vice versa. He becomes able to prolong the sex act at will and capable of holding a relaxed, timeless space that supports woman (and thereby himself) as an equal and opposite force in experiencing orgasmic fulfillment.

When man and woman are rooted in nature—man as dynamic force, woman as receptive force—there is an intrinsic movement as a by-product of the meeting of opposite polarities. Spontaneous, inherent circles of giving and receiving come into play. Man gives to woman, she receives from man; woman gives to man, he receives from woman. Many men have probably experienced, however briefly, no greater blessing than being the recipient of woman's love; there is nothing more gratifying or significant in the life of a man. When he receives a shower of female essence, divine feminine nectar, the pure sweetness of it is a magically empowering experience for a man. It is the love that is awakened in her through the power of a loving penis. Such enchanting experiences are the true outcome of sexual union, but happen much too seldom. Normally at the outset of a relationship, when the situation is fresh and new, magical experiences naturally occur. The knack is to keep re-creating the newness and not fall into habit or take each other for granted.

SEXUAL CONDITIONING INFLUENCES SEXUAL BEHAVIOR

Very few men have conscious control over themselves or their penises in sex, which puts them at a disadvantage in creating love. Lack of control exists because there is a complete absence of constructive information. Instead, unconscious impressions about sex from earliest childhood accumulate and shape the individual, gradually forming a sexual conditioning that distorts the individual's natural sexual responses or expression.

Although clarification about sex, or useful sex education, is virtually nonexistent in our culture, sex continues to be a driving and distracting force. But at the same time this powerful force is kept under wraps, like a secret. Most people are involved in sex in some way, but nobody acknowledges it, shares information, or even talks about it. Sex shifts away from the body and becomes an aspect of the mind as expressed in thoughts, fantasies, dreams, and voyeurism, and this is true even in self-pleasuring. Sex leaves the realm of the humanly sensitive flesh to become something you think about a zillion times more than you actually do.

When a man finally gets together with a woman, he operates on his accumulated past experiences and guesswork, and hopes for the best. Beneath multiple layers of bravado and performance frequently lies a sexual insecurity that gnaws away at the depths of his being. Such tension will exacerbate any other presexual tension, causing the man to perhaps feel out of control, especially concerning ejaculation.

Correspondence between the Penis and the Vagina

To shift to a higher realm of sexual experience a man has to reevaluate his penis and the way he uses it inside the vagina. He must use his penis with intelligence, maturity, and vision.

Nature intended the penis to operate as a highly sensitive, perceptive magnetic instrument. Although the penis and vagina are physical organs, they are designed to communicate on a refined energy level. The entire penis is a channel, a conduit through which life force moves from man into woman. Woman receives this force and draws it into herself. The response or communication between the genitals can first be felt as a vibrant sensation of aliveness on a fine cellular level. When we are caught up in sexual doing, there is no opportunity to relax and simply be in the body and experience this subtle vitality. When mechanical movements cease, we can begin to tune in to a finer level of sensitivity and delicate sensation.

The vagina and penis as equal and opposite forces are designed by nature for a "happening." When one fits into the other, man can begin to experience emanations from his penis, like electromagnetic streamings, that become increasingly ecstatic as they spread throughout the body. By developing an inner listening to—and with—his penis and genital region, his overall approach to making love will become more sensitive and conscious.

DEVELOPING SENSITIVITY
THROUGH BEING CONSCIOUS

When a man begins to make love with awareness and experiment with stillness, he may be surprised to notice a relative absence of sensitivity in his penis. Without the familiar stimulation and intensity, it's not so easy for him to find a real inner connection to his genital area. Such lack of sensitivity is to be expected after many years of tense, goal-oriented sex. The good news is that sensitivity will quickly return to the penis through a relaxed style of lovemaking.

On the eighth and final day of our workshops we usually ask the men, "Does your penis now feel more sensitive?" Virtually all raise their hands to confirm a dramatic increase in sensitivity. By reducing the friction movements—the doing—they are able to redirect their attention to an inner awareness of the penis and its vitality. Even men who have used the penis in another way for forty or fifty years notice a change in sensitivity and aliveness within just a few days. The body's regenerative power under conducive conditions is extraordinary. There exists an intrinsic drive toward purity and wholeness when the intelligence of the body is embraced.

Using the Imagination

If you lack sensitivity in the penis when there is no movement or stimulation, your creative imagination can help your body to cooperate with your inner reality. Imagination can be a powerful tool for awakening an inner, cellular experience. You can take your attention into the penis and visualize it as a channel for potency, warmth, love, light, gold, or whatever encourages an inner perception and flow. Energy follows imagination, so by leading the way with visualization, you can actually begin to experience vitality and sensation.

We know how well the imagination works in sexual fantasy, but in that situation we are imagining something that doesn't exist, so we are completely absent and disconnected from what is happening in the here and now. When imagination is directed toward something that actually exists in the energetic realm, it has the power to elevate the experience and gradually open man to the inner experience of his radiant penis.

Bringing Attention from the Head to the Perineum

Generally speaking a man will tend to have most of his attention on the head of the penis, naturally, because this is where he experiences the most intense pleasure. To begin to shift attention away from the head of the penis, visualize your penis as a channel for potency, warmth, and love. Imagine that it is a fountain of light and liquid gold energy, circulating its dynamic force back into your body. Envision your penis as a channel or conduit, and refocus your attention on the base of your penis, in the area of the perineum. The perineum, a small, coin-sized area of knotty muscle lying directly in front of the anus, is virtually the root of the penis and is its energetic source. It is where the muscles and tissues that form the penis initially emerge from the floor of your pelvis.

When you begin to make love and feel the sexual heat rising, bring your attention to the perineum. Consciously relax the entire pelvic floor area, including the anus and testicles. When you notice your attention start to drift—there are, after all, abundant distractions—you may notice that in your absence the pelvic floor area once again contracts and tightens. Relaxing the anus frequently and maintaining awareness of the base of the penis will give you an inner feeling of your penis as a complete unit, rather than a disembodied tool for thrusting. It becomes a divine instrument capable of channeling subtle energies that flow or stream from the root upward to the radiant head, and beyond into your receptive partner. Be aware of your breathing and of the subtle sensations deep within your physical core as your inner rod of magnetism awakens. Notice how the life force rises to caress your heart into vibrant aliveness. (See the appendix at the back of the book for specific ways to increase sensitivity.)

A HIGHLY SENSITIVE MAGNET

The silky, slippery, smooth, sensitive head of the penis bears testament to its powerful magnetic properties. The head radiates life force, energy, and potency, which correspond directly with the receptive, relaxed, inviting vaginal environment. The head of the penis also acts as a catalyst with profoundly healing properties (see chapter 8 on sexual healing and male authority). When the head of the penis corresponds to its equal and opposite pole, the connection is able to generate states of ecstasy. Tantra master Barry Long, from Australia, says that a man should attempt to "become" his penis while making love. Through awareness and presence a man can gradually learn to merge with his penis, and be his penis.

There is a ruthless emphasis in our culture on the size of a man's penis when erect, and even when it is flaccid. Sometimes the two don't even correlate, since it's impossible to estimate the erect size of a penis based on its flaccid state. Convention insists that bigger is better, so a man may have feelings of shame or insecurity because of his size, which affects his capacity to trust, love, and value his own penis.

In the tantric approach, sensitivity and capacity of presence are more important than size and performance. It is true that a bigger penis is able to cause more friction in the vagina, but a penis that is big and hard can also be numb and insensitive in itself, as well as cause discomfort to a woman. However, when there is a shift in our thinking about sex, we can begin to give value to our subtle energy exchanges, which means that any size is perfect. Many men discover that their optimally perceptive sensitive state is when the penis is only half erect. How you do something is much more meaningful than what you do, or the size or rigidity of your sex organ. The penis is innately intelligent, and if man is able to relax back into himself, nature will express itself through him.

PERSONAL SHARING
Focusing on the Inner Body

During the lovemaking retreat we repeated one exercise several times, which involved closing my eyes and focusing just on the inner body (the home in my body) in order to feel a connection with my pelvis. It was always a beautiful experience for me.

When I felt connected with myself, I slowly opened my eyes, still focusing on the inside, and slowly turned to my partner, who had just done the same exercise. While slowly coming together in this manner, I was full of joy and love. I realized that my penis stiffened and I wanted to share this pleasant feeling with my partner and rub my penis against her, as I used to in the past.

However, this time I tried something new. I stayed with my feeling, sensed my penis from inside, and experienced a strange energy filling my body and rising to my heart. This wonderful connection, this streaming of energy from my penis to my heart, was very fulfilling for me and left a deep impression. All this happened just because I was alert and contained my feeling, and did not automatically project my feeling out of my own body.

PERSONAL SHARING
Swaying in a Tantric Dance

One sensation that came up again and again was of a kind of dance happening between penis and vagina. When I was inside my wife, I perceived a soft motion between us—like leaves swaying gently in a warm breeze, or as if my penis were surrounded by soft, warm liquid. Although seen from an outside perspective our bodies did not move, my motions were, in fact, in harmony with her motions, and I felt deeply connected to my beloved in what felt like a dance between the female and the male. As I remember this event, I wonder again about the untapped potential of our sexual organs. Tantra is a true adventure to me. My perceptions during lovemaking have become more refined, diversified, and intense. This makes lovemaking more touching, colorful, and deeply conscious for me, both physically and energetically.

I have a beautiful experience to share: One morning when we were making love and were inside of each other, I felt as if my penis were surrounded by warm liquid honey. My wife's vagina was soft and receptive, I was very present and focused, and a common space formed between us, a healing space in which my masculinity encountered the femininity of my beloved. Energetically there was just this one space, within which we could love each other in total freedom. After some time we changed position, and my wife suddenly got aroused and had an orgasm. After that her vagina felt tense and tight, and the space between us had disappeared.

PERSONAL SHARING
One with Myself and with My Lover

I've begun to notice the ability of my penis to stay erect without my being aroused. Previously erectness was inextricably connected with arousal. I happen to see a sexy woman, and poing—my penis gets stiff. My wife touches my penis—poing. But now the poing happens without any arousal, but only if we are inside of each other and I am present, focused, and relaxed. There are two factors that make it extra easy: If my lover is also present and if I am deeply in her vagina. Most of those times I feel a strong energy flow within myself and between us. Everything around us becomes unimportant, and I am one with myself and my lover. I feel held, loved, and simply at home in myself and in everything that is.

Tantric Inspiration

Remain with the beginning; do not move to the end. How to remain in the beginning? Many things are to be remembered. First, don't take the sex act as a way of going anywhere. Don't take it as a means: it is the end in itself. There is no end to it; it is not a means. Secondly, do not think of the future; remain with the present. And if you cannot remain in the present in the beginning part of the sex act, then you can never remain in the present—because the very nature of the act is such that you are thrown into the present.

Remain in the present. Enjoy the meeting of two bodies, two souls, and merge into each other, melt into each other. Forget that you are going anywhere. Remain in the moment going nowhere, and melt. Warmth, love, should be made a situation for two persons to melt into each other. That is why, if there is no love, the sex act is a hurried act. You are using the other; the other is just a means. And the other is using you. You are exploiting each other, not merging into each other. With love you can merge. This merging in the beginning will give you many new insights.

If you are not in a hurry to finish the act, the act, by and by, becomes less and less sexual and more and more spiritual. Sex organs also melt into each other. A deep silent communion happens between two body energies, and then you can remain for hours together. This togetherness moves deeper and deeper as time passes. But don't think. Remain with the moment deeply merged. It becomes an ecstasy, a *samadhi,* cosmic consciousness. And if you can know this, if you can feel and realize this, your sexual mind will become nonsexual.

OSHO, TRANSCRIBED TEACHINGS,
VIGYAN BHAIRAV TANTRA

6

AWARENESS, MOVEMENT, PENETRATION, AND ERECTION

AWARENESS

The expression "It's not what you do, but how you do it" is more deeply understood through these simple yet profound words of Osho: "Tantra is the transformation of sex into love through awareness." These few words encapsulate the essence of tantra, which is about awareness—nothing more, nothing less. If we are aware and conscious during sex, sex transforms into love. Awareness changes the whole quality of sex, and the fragrance and climate of love is naturally generated through awareness. Woman's heart and body respond vibrantly to man rooted in the present through his awareness.

Staying Present within the Body
The elusive present moment is created through bringing awareness to the body, holding the attention in the body, millisecond by millisecond.

Being aware of body position, movements, and breath and relaxing habitual tensions are basic tools to accessing and staying in the present. The body always exists in the present; it is the mind that roams around in past and future thoughts. Before a man can understand how to remain present while making love with a woman, he must first establish a relationship with his own body. He can literally embody his own body by taking his attention inside the body and away from thoughts and fantasies. As one retreat participant a few years ago reported, "It's incredible, I am a fifty-four-year-old man, and nobody has ever told me to feel inside my body. And it is paradise in there!"

Another encouraging example was this: less than twenty-four hours into the retreat a man raised his hand and complained, "It's all very well for you to say, 'Feel all the subtle pleasant inner sensations.' You've been doing it for more than twenty years. I can feel absolutely nothing." We assured him that he needed to give himself more time and that practice makes perfect. The week continued without any further comment from him, so on the final day we asked how he was feeling in his body. He looked at us, eyes and face radiant with love, and said just one word: "Unbelievable!"

See the appendix for specific exercises to bring attention into your body.

Relax and Breathe

There is a tendency for us to tighten various muscles or clench muscle groups unconsciously, without really realizing it. Such tensions have become a habit and a way of life to the extent that as we are falling asleep, we may realize we are unconsciously holding ourselves up on the bed. We are not letting go and allowing even our place of comfort and repose to fully receive us. Physical tensions compress the energy system and restrict the expansion of vitality through the body. So it is enormously helpful to become aware of these tensions and release them, or breathe into them, while you are making love. Physical relaxation and conscious breathing will also reduce the pressure to ejaculate. (See the appendix for particular ways to scan the body and check for tension.)

Eye Contact and Communication

Generally speaking people make love in the dark, with closed eyes and without much meeting of the eyes. Although it might feel a little awkward in the beginning, connecting eye to eye immediately creates a feeling of intimacy and brings you in touch with the present. The eye contact is not a fixed stare, but an introverted, soft, receptive gaze that invites your partner into you. As you enter woman, or as you change positions, allow the eyes to meet and engage. And at the same time, feel how your genitals engage. Maintaining eye contact is not a rule but a suggestion, a tool to increase awareness and presence. Closing the eyes and taking awareness into your own body, in order to strengthen your inner connection and sensitivity, will also be necessary from time to time. It's a good thing to tell your partner why you are closing your eyes, so the person doesn't feel abandoned or excluded.

To amplify the experience of the present moment, you will be surprised how much sharing what is happening to you on an inner body level—communicating out loud—helps to intensify the inner experience. Acknowledging your inner sensitivities and sensations verbally has the effect of intensifying them, and you'll find your body unexpectedly rewarding you for having noticed the existence of its cellular subtle ties and vitality. Only a few words are needed to convey what you feel within yourself on a body-heart-soul level, as if you are giving an inner weather report. Your partner does not have to respond directly, unless she wants to communicate what she feels within herself. These kinds of body reports are a great key to tracking your way to the present and can be done either before as a kind of foreplay or while actually making love. It will also eliminate any need for the clichéd, "Was it good for you?" because you will know during the process.

Consideration of the Receptive Force

As we now can appreciate, there is a distinct advantage to the female partner being in a state of receptivity in order to allow the male force through her. Like man, woman also needs the opportunity to enter her own body and become alive to her inner world. Since you know it will take longer for woman's body to warm up, wait until your woman says she is ready to take you in. Wait for a "yes," an invitation. Women tend to yield to pressure because they have not yet learned to trust and honor their feminine systems. They get messages from their bodies, but there is a tendency for woman to override her inner wisdom; frequently she feels compelled to let man into her before she is truly ready. Part of woman's sexual conditioning is to please man, usually because she is afraid of losing him or losing his love. When man is aware of the pleasing tendency of woman, he can begin to understand it as the female counterpart to the male pressure to perform.

When you wait, create space, and support woman to relax into herself and connect with her internal world, she opens with ease and enthusiasm. Man creates the potential to be inside woman endlessly and tap her higher orgasmic energies. When a "yes" comes from woman in her totality, it is as if she's plugged into a circuit from which she finds it difficult to disconnect. She is neither frigid nor rigid, but vital and receptive. For man to be a channel or conduit for his true male energy, the equal and opposite force must also be available, so man needs to be constantly aware of the receptacle that is receiving the flow of his life force.

MOVEMENT

There is a common misconception that tantra means no movement during sex. We heartily endorse movement, not for the sake of movement itself, but because it creates more aliveness and presence.

Movements should also seek to enhance the correspondent dynamic-receptive potential of the genital contact. Stillness is an option, and something that you may develop an appreciation for over time, but initially most people usually enjoy alternating phases of movement with phases of stillness.

Awareness and Tempo

Any movement done consciously, which means you feel yourself as you do it, changes the quality of the experience dramatically. Done with awareness, all movements naturally become slower, and the body becomes more sensual and sensitive; you become totally engaged in the unfolding present. Be alert and aware as you approach each other, embrace, kiss, move, change position, move the penis within the vagina—be aware in whatever you do. There is a natural slowing down when any action is done with awareness. You are not slowing down to follow a rule, but instead discovering that when you are aware, you do in fact move more slowly. And you can feel more; your sensitivity increases. Slowness is an outcome, a by-product of being more conscious. Out of curiosity or for fun, you can ask yourself, "How slow is slow?" And get into an inquiry.

Come together in an unhurried way, while staying in awareness. Remain alert, attentive, and conscious in the body. Let there be a flow; allow it to happen, rather than forcing or pushing it in certain directions. Allow an easy, innocent, playful, spontaneous unfolding without knowing what will happen next.

Goal-oriented Movement Becomes Mechanical

Movements that have the goal of building up to a climax will have an intrinsic pressure powering them, whereas movements that do not have a goal can arise fluidly from the requirements of bodies in the moment. There is nothing wrong with movement per se; movement is life, but at the same time we need to remain aware and steer clear of the tendency to be mechanical in the sex act. The usual movement of the penis in the vagina is forward and backward thrusts, a linear movement. But movements can also be made in a more expansive three-dimensional way, reaching into different angles of the vaginal canal (as described later, in chapter 8 within the context of sexual healing and male empowerment).

Movements made with the intention of creating pleasure and excitement will tend to become mechanical, and when we become like machines, we lose awareness and sensitivity. With the focus on stimulation, our awareness of what is taking place in the body on a more subtle level tends to diminish. Our attention or focus is more on building up intensity, rather than on taking delight in each of the individual movements taking place.

Usually, a woman will push her genitals forward (using her pelvis) at the very same moment the man thrusts or moves into her. Physically speaking, just from the mechanics of the musculature, the vagina becomes narrower and tighter during a forward push. This tightening results in the vagina being less receptive in this phase of the movement. As a consequence, woman is not truly available to the dynamic force entering her body.

Another option is to let man do the moving, while woman holds still. Instead of woman pushing forward to meet man's movement, she tilts her pelvis upward at an angle and remains still. In this nonmoving position a woman is able to put all her attention into her vagina—into the receiving, absorbing, and welcoming of the penis into her body. A pillow can be placed beneath the buttocks in order to raise the level of the pelvis, if so desired. Man will perceive his conscious movement in woman far more deeply if she is able to fulfill her part of the design, which is to act as receptor for the dynamic force.

The Difference between Lust and Passion

When the dynamic and receptive forces in our bodies are honored, we become more present and naturally more passionate. Passion is pure presence, aliveness, and spontaneity. In passion there can also be strong movements that might look the same as the movements of conventional sex from the outside, but the inner experience is vastly different. The movements contain an inner stillness because they belong to the domain of the here and now; there is no direction, no goal, and no agenda. Nothing is planned or expected. Instead, each individual is engaged, with full awareness merged into the unfolding of each and every millimeter of movement. Each millisecond of any movement is a completion in itself.

In contrast, when movement contains lust, there is a tendency to be ahead of oneself, slightly mechanical, with the movements being focused on building up to a crescendo. The individual movements are not independent or complete in themselves. When lust drives the lovemaking, frustration and disappointment are likely to follow a sudden interruption because something desired was not reached or achieved. The act is incomplete because the goal was not fulfilled. By contrast, when passion is unexpectedly interrupted, everything is simply perfect as it is. Each second has been utterly complete in itself, so there is simply no sense of any loss at all. In fact, passionate sex can be resumed at any moment, while in lustful sex there will usually be a sense of deflation and loss of interest because the heat and excitement will have gone out of the situation.

THE ART OF CONSCIOUS PENETRATION

When erection is present it is recommended that the very first movement into the vagina be exceptionally conscious. The first move sets the stage for what is to follow. The penis should enter the vagina slowly, millimeter by millimeter. A number of positions are possible, the most direct and easy being the missionary position, with woman lying on her back and man kneeling between her legs. The head of the penis can enter the vagina and gradually open it along its entire length, gently probing slowly but surely up the canal. Resting from time to time allows you to take in the view, which means feeling in and down into your body and especially into your penis. A single movement can easily be extended to many minutes, or an entire lovemaking session of several hours can be one divine immersion in woman's body. These experiences can change your life and your whole view of sex.

The problem with an entry by the penis that is fast or aggressive and lacking in awareness is that woman (unconsciously or consciously) closes her vagina to protect herself from possible intense pain. The upper vagina tightens to prevent the penis from thrusting into the very delicate and sensitive cervix—the entrance to the womb. When woman is hit here it really hurts. Such naturally defensive contractions, both physical and psychological, definitely influence woman's receptivity and capacity to absorb, which means she is no longer feminine in relation to man. With conscious, slow penetration, woman has the chance to invite, welcome, and caress each millimeter of the probing penis.

There is a distinction between being careful and being conscious. One is not being "careful" in relation to woman; carefulness implies a certain tension, a holding back, a fear of hurting the other, which is more an attitude lacking in self-awareness. With carefulness, one's attention is externally focused on the other and not on the self. We are up and out, and have left home, so to speak. When one is conscious, one is self-aware and automatically acts with care as a by-product of that awareness, rather than as an intention to "be careful." When a man is conscious, he also becomes more confident.

Awareness, Slowness, and Sensitivity

The greatest advantage of awareness, of being conscious during penetration, is that you can feel "into" the penis on a cellular level. Finally you have the time and there is nowhere to go (toward ejaculation), so you can instead focus your attention inside the penis itself. Listening to the penis and becoming aware of its gradual movement greatly increases its sensitivity and allows the perception of inner, fine, cellular, delicate, delightful sensations that expand throughout the body. An unhurried, aimless, no goals approach is vital to making this possible.

Ecstatic, thrilling, touching experiences occur through a correspondence of opposites. In fitting snugly together with sustained contact, penis and vagina respond to each other according to an innate intelligence. The penis is a powerful instrument able to generate divine states of ecstasy when arriving in its truly complementary environment.

Deep, Sustained Penetration

As a general orientation, when there is erection and the possibility of gradual, sensitive penetration, the penetration should be sustained in the depths of the vagina. (This subject is also dealt with in chapter 8 on sexual healing and male authority. Both chapters should be read in order to grasp the full implications of remaining deep inside woman.) This means that when you eventually arrive (after the minutes given to the first journey down the canal), you remain with the penis inside, resting in the depths, and do not immediately withdraw in order to repeat the movement. Instead, take the time to intentionally bring your entire awareness into the penis and "be" your penis, attempting to sense the tissues from within, to merge and melt with them. You do not force your penis into woman, but you force your awareness, your point of attention, into your penis, remaining at the same time relaxed and observing. These are two very different experiences for both parties involved.

At the end of the vagina lies the extremely sensitive cervix; and as already mentioned, it can be indescribably painful if the penis head aggressively hits this spot, so it is important to arrive here with sensitivity. When you arrive at the end of the canal or as far as you can go or whenever you have the feeling that the penis head is pushing into the walls with pressure anywhere along the way, it's very important to drop back a hairsbreadth or two. This minute fraction of space removes any pressure and intention, and creates "breathing room" for the "porous" contact that is required for an energy exchange. When the push is purely physical and hard, the vaginal cells withdraw and close in response. When the contact is subtle, gentle, easy, and spacious, the cells are able to relax and open. Sometimes during penetration the penis will encounter pains held in the vagina, a topic that will be covered specifically in chapter 8 on sexual healing, along with diagrams of suitable positions for deep, sustained penetration.

Lubrication—the Secret of Sensual Penetration

A slippery, smooth, silky, slow, sensual penetration simply has to be one of life's greatest joys, for both man and woman. Use lubricant without hesitation and with pleasure, and use it every time. Oil the penis, the vaginal lips, and the entrance. It's a great part of foreplay, especially when woman does the oiling. Oil was used by Taoists thousands of years ago and is said to reduce bacteria levels in the vagina. Use thin, fragrance-free vegetable oil, such as almond oil. It is also suggested that woman hold her lips/labia open when man is about to enter her. Using both hands, she clears the entrance from any obstructing skin folds and holds her hands in position for a while. This assistance guarantees a smooth, pleasurable journey.

Vaginal Dryness

Without high levels of stimulation woman is less likely to become "wet," which is quite normal. Also, when women approach menopause and suffer from dryness, penetration can become difficult, painful, or impossible. With a slow, conscious, oily penis, miracles are possible. Women who have not been able to make love for years are able to get back into it with ease. Gradually, in time, the vaginal tissues relax, regenerate, and naturally become more moist.

Condoms

Condoms are sometimes necessary for contraception or health reasons, and are without doubt a layer between man and his sensitivity. However, according to people who have used them and our own personal experience, man is capable of feeling the delicate, subtle, electromagnetic exchange through condoms. The basic sensitivity is not seriously affected or compromised.

If condoms are used, don't use oil as a lubricant; oil destroys rubber and compromises contraception. Use only water-based gels, which can be obtained from a pharmacy. This is a good moment to stress the importance of genital hygiene and daily cleansing of the penis, particularly underneath the foreskin.

While on the subject of contraception, it is important to acknowledge here that a woman responds to sexual invitations much more readily if there is no fear of pregnancy. Such fear can definitely contribute to a woman's reluctance or lack of availability during her fertile years. If man is willing to take responsibility for contraception, either in taking care of himself or supporting his woman to take the appropriate care in the moment and not in theory, he is helping himself enormously. Some men choose the option of a vasectomy as a solution for contraception, and from time to time we receive queries asking if vasectomy disturbs male potency. We can say with confidence that vasectomy does not appear to affect male potency and may even increase potency, in that it allows woman to be more free with herself. Relieved of concerns about conception, she can be more spontaneous and may also wish to make love with greater frequency.

Soft Penetration—Entry without Erection

Soft entry is a pure and simple alternative when there is no erection. It completely eliminates the pressure of having to have an erection in order to have sex. Given the general lack of stimulation, not having an erection is quite normal and nothing to be concerned about. Soft entry actually bypasses many erection concerns and issues, and gives us a humble, human way to get our bodies together. The advantage of a soft start is that both man and woman begin at zero, so to speak, allowing their temperatures to warm up together. Soft entry is very easy and, with practice, can happen in the flash of a second. There are two possibilities: man puts his penis inside woman, or woman puts the penis inside her. We recommend the second option.

Man Initiates Soft Penetration

Man kneels between woman's open legs, as seen in figure 6.1. Woman can place a flat, firm cushion underneath her buttocks. The lifted position raises the level of the pelvis and brings the vagina closer to the penis. Woman holds her labia open, as described earlier, and man introduces the head of the penis into the entrance of the vagina using his fingers. Push the head in a little bit (be sure your fingernails are trimmed), move the fingers back a few centimeters, and insert the penis a little further into the vagina. Step by step, wiggle and walk the penis inside the entrance.

When the penis is in the vagina as far as you can manage (even the head is a good start), remain kneeling and bring the pelvises together. Or lower yourself down on top of your partner, holding yourself up with your arms. Or lie forward on your partner and then roll onto your sides, man remaining between woman's legs.

Woman Initiates Soft Entry

The easiest and most comfortable position for soft penetration is the side position called scissors, because of the scissor-like interlacing of the legs. The advantage of the scissors position is that nobody is on top and nobody is underneath, which is indeed very relaxing. Man is on his side, while woman is lying on her back with her legs inserted, scissors fashion, between man's legs. You can stay in this position for several hours quite easily. From scissors position any number of other positions can be reached, which will be elaborated on in chapter 7.

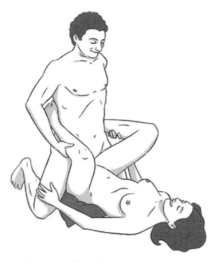

Fig. 6.1. This figure shows man in
the middle position suitable for soft entry

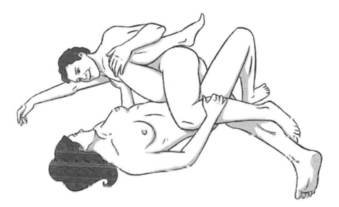

Fig. 6.2. The scissors position for soft penetration

Bring your legs together, as shown in figure 6.2. The scissors position can be assumed from either man's left side or his right side, and it's a good idea to change sides regularly to avoid getting habituated (and therefore less alert) to one side only. Woman opens her legs, opens her labia, and then reaches for the penis, which has been oiled in advance. By now it's probably not so soft, so the entering is made even easier.

The first two fingers of one hand (short nails so as not to scratch the vagina) are put behind the head of the penis and squeezed firmly to get a grip (see fig. 6.3). The same two fingers on the other hand can stabilize the penis at the base. Woman pulls the head toward the vagina and inserts it in the entrance. Fingers are moved back a few centimeters, then gradually walked step-by-step into the vagina. At first the head may be as far as it gets, but with practice, it does get perfect. Woman must avoid looking between her legs during this delicate operation because the tightening of her abdominal muscles (needed to lift up the head to look) will also tighten the vagina and make penetration difficult, if not impossible. Looking is fine as you get set up, but then lie back and relax before you initiate the insertion.

Then move the pelvises together, joining firmly in connection. If by any chance man rolls back slightly—which pulls the penis out—wedge a flat pillow from behind, under his pelvis/buttocks. The pillow wedge tilts man's body forward slightly and stabilizes the position. Pillows can be used for support wherever needed, for instance, under the calf/knee of man's upper leg. This also reduces the weight on woman's body, as well as giving man a floating feeling. Be sure to get yourselves as comfortable as possible so that your systems can relax. Small discomforts can be distractions, and instead of delighting in your inner pleasures, you tune in to your lack of comfort.

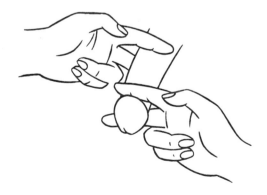

Fig. 6.3. Woman's finger position behind penis head

SPONTANEOUS ERECTION
AND IMPOTENCE

Spontaneous erection within the vagina is not something that can be expected or demanded of the body. It is a by-product of a special constellation of factors, among which are awareness, presence, relaxation, and love.

Erection Responsibility Is Shared

Until now, whether he likes it or not, erection has been considered man's job, which has been a big part of his performance pressure. Conventionally, erection usually depends on stimulation and excitement, and many anxieties or fears about erection can cause a disturbance in the psyche, perhaps becoming expressed in distorted ways.

As a partnership continues, a man can easily experience a lack of erection because of a lack of excitement. The woman is known, the situation is known, and the routine is known, so there is nothing to get him really excited. However, with a new vision of sex we realize that excitement is not necessarily a basic ingredient of the sexual experience.

Erection is definitely possible without stimulation and excitement when a man begins to trust his penis. A true erection is an electromagnetic response to the equal and opposite force exerted by the vagina. From a soft state, the penis can slowly rise as a direct response to the vagina surrounding it. The female force plays an equal role; through receptivity it starts to "draw" and effectively pulls the penis into an erection, millimeter by millimeter. The penis unfolds like a slow snake winding upward in a circular spiraling motion. Erection without stimulation or excitement can also happen when in close proximity to a woman. The female force exerts an influence on the male force without your actually being inside her. Men say that it is as if the penis awakens in the atmosphere of love created through presence and awareness

A spontaneous erection is one that arises out of the moment, due to the polarity between dynamic and receptive forces and the presence two people bring into the situation. Erections that arise spontaneously do not require stimulation or fantasy to keep them going; they simply need presence and awareness. The instant one person's attention wavers, the penis starts to wind back down, coiling like a snake. Quickly retrieving one's presence and releasing distracting thoughts will cause the erection to grow again. The penis is capable of performing a snake dance within woman—a miraculous experience for any man.

Lack of Sensitivity

The first few times soft penetration is tried, most men will find that they do not "feel" much in their penises (as mentioned earlier). This is very common and will change as soon as the penis adjusts to a new way of being used and perceived by man. This insensitivity is due to a long history of stimulation, so for it to be a little numb is not really surprising. The way to retrieve sensitivity is to relax into woman, spend as much time inside her as possible, and take full consciousness down into your penis. Begin to "be" inside the penis, treat it with love, and gradually sensitivity will return.

Usually the woman is able to feel your penis, even if you cannot perceive it. She is usually very content with soft penetration and the experience of subtle, ecstatic emanations from the penis. It is a great support to the man if a woman can communicate what she feels within herself (her inner sensitivity) out loud in words while making love, particularly in the situation where a man discovers he is not (yet) able to feel the power residing within his own penis. At the very least, it's relaxing to know that woman can feel man, even if he cannot feel himself. And she, as container, is bound to be more perceptive initially.

Impotence Issues

Impotence—lack of erection—is a deep-seated fear in most men, provoking anxiety at an almost primal level. Excitement leads to a certain type of erection that is very fragile and requires stimulation to keep it going. Impotence is no longer an issue when soft entry used. And—surprise, surprise—erection may take place on its own. The best cure for impotence is to keep putting yourself in the situation and continue making love with no erection. In time things are highly likely to change as sensitivity returns.

Several years ago a man with an inherited erectile dysfunction came to our group with his wife. He had been using penis implants up until this point and was wondering whether to drop the implant and instead try the way we had been explaining during the group. His success has been incredible. He does not have full erections now, but enough that it is no longer a problem. He describes his experience below.

PERSONAL SHARING
From Impotence to Daily Lovemaking

First of all, we bought your new book, Tantric Love—Feeling versus Emotion: Golden Rules to Make Love Easy *(the German edition). My wife read it within three hours. I took more time, but also read it quite quickly. We can confirm all that you have been saying. Emotions and feelings are too often mixed up, and very few people are aware of this important difference. (See chapter 9 for more on the distinction between feelings and emotions.)*

Last December we attended a workshop for Vipassana meditation. The theme was arrogance; the solution is humility. The insight and the teaching was: Our minds are constantly using our senses to compare all our perceptions and assess them as positive/good (I want more), negative/harmful (I want to get rid of it), or equal/good (which is not really satisfactory either). As long as we constantly compare, we are never relaxed in life and are unable to enjoy a love relationship with awareness and equanimity.

It lines up perfectly with your explanation of why there is so much incomprehension and jealousy between couples. In any event, we learned that making love your way takes away so much of the pressure that many reasons for comparison vanish, and disappointment (emotions) within yourself and against your partner just doesn't manifest. For us making love has become a kind of meditation, combining intimacy with spirituality, which we consider the whipped cream on the cake.

But let us tell you what happened to us since we attended the course with you a second time. After the first course with you a few years ago we practiced love within my almost nonexistent erection capability (owing to my medical condition). In the beginning we made love two to three times a week, and slowly cut back to making love once a week, keeping this frequency stable. We noted that regardless of the unhurried and relaxed way of making love, there was often the feeling that after almost an entire week it was about time to have sex together, and this created increasingly unpleasant pressure to perform.

After the first course, my wife started paying a lot of attention to my penis, massaging me and holding my penis in her hand every night when we went to bed, falling asleep this way. My penis got so much attention that it started to react to her contact, not with an erection, but with a kind of aliveness. It swells up just enough that I can introduce it into her vagina without great effort, and is also firm enough to go for an ejaculation, if I so desire. Even if my penis extends less than four inches, it is good enough to have the real feeling of having sex. Since my wife has never had an orgasm by penetration, but only by stimulation of her clitoris, this "handicap" of my shortened penis is not really bothering us. Sometimes I feel that I'm not a "real man with a hard one," but the sexual satisfaction I experience with my wife vastly exceeds the short event of conventional sex and ejaculation.

After our second course with you we both had the impulse to say, "Why don't we decide to have sex every day to get rid of the pressure of having to do it after a number of days? Let's create an atmosphere in which making love daily is as normal as eating meals." We decided to connect our genitals every morning at daybreak. We set the clock one hour earlier in the morning and start with twenty minutes of cuddling and caressing each other. Then my wife celebrates the oil ceremony, oiling her vagina and giving a short oil massage to my penis—just enough for it to be gently hard and easily introduced into her vagina. We remain connected for another twenty minutes, and then either turn and change position or share some moments of in and out movements. About once a week one of us—or both—feels like going for an orgasm, and we celebrate it without restriction. Finally we have another twenty minutes of cuddling—relaxing, drowsing, caressing, and so on. After an hour we get up, my wife takes a shower, and I sit down for Vipassana meditation till she is ready to leave the house for work. Often our genitals radiate pleasant vibrations and pulsate throughout our entire bodies for the whole day. It is just gorgeous.

We started this a few months ago, and since then have hardly missed a day of making love. It has become so natural and uncomplicated that we actually long for it if we have to miss one day. Our entire relationship has reached another level because we can behave so freely and openly, which I never before thought possible.

Sometimes we look back and ask ourselves what triggered our starting to insist on making love every day. We don't know, really, it just clicked and we knew we wanted to try it. During our second course with you we heard from a couple resolutely doing a fifteen-minute tantric get together every morning who seemed to be happy and united, so maybe this was the final kick for us to start.

We are very thankful for having met you and having been able to learn this method of making love from you. In my special situation with a medical condition, I often wonder what I would have done after conventional sex was no longer possible for me. I don't even want to imagine.

PERSONAL SHARING
Viagra Is No Longer Necessary

Since puberty, erection has been of great importance for me. The first time I had sex with a woman it happened in a very small compact car, and

I had no idea where to put my long legs. Due to the excitement, I did not find my way into her vagina and had a premature ejaculation. Ever since, ejaculation and penetration were stressful for me. Each time I met a new woman, I immediately had a fear of failure and thus, difficulty with the erection. It wasn't until my first longer partnership that this theme began to lose its importance.

My penultimate partnership was very much affected by wild sex and strong emotions. It was sex that glued us together and helped us to come together again and again, but in the end, even sex did not work any more. This resulted in new emotions, mutual hurt, and finally, in separation. Since I was nearing the end of my fifties at that time I presumed that sex was over for me, until I found out about the remedy for erections: Cialis (Viagra). I was very relieved to be able to have sexual contact with new women, and realized that I retained my capacity for erection even beyond the action time of the remedy. This also showed me the psychological aspect of the erection deficit. When I met my new wife, we had a weekend relationship for the first two years. I got used to taking Cialis each time before we met, because it gave me a sense of security. When we took a two-week vacation, one pill at the beginning of the holiday was enough.

After we read your book, The Heart of Tantric Sex, my wife didn't want me to take the remedy any more, so I promised to take it only after having talked to her. At home, where we were already comfortable with the relaxed way of lovemaking, I found taking it less and less necessary.

Before the lovemaking retreat we had not seen each other for three weeks. During the first three days of the seminar, I again experienced some pressure with the issues, and had trouble keeping my sense of humor about erection and penetration. I feared that since I was sixty-three years old, my virility was definitely over, so I told her that I would like to take Viagra again. When she declined my request, we had a talk with the two of you and somehow I relaxed after having talked about it so openly. The loving *support of my partner, and the length of time that we took for lovemaking, has resulted ever since in much heartfelt and relaxed sex. I learned that even with a weak erection at the beginning, lovemaking lasted longer, and was heartfelt and deep. Our love grew and I was able to relax more and more deeply. Since then our love and our sexuality have reached a new dimension. For me it has been a gift. Being able to let go of goal-oriented male sexuality as my erection was getting weaker has caused our love to grow. Thank you both for this wonderful experience.*

PERSONAL SHARING
My Body Keeps Me Honest

During lovemaking, my body lets me know if I am touching from my heart. I became aware of it when I was lying in bed with my wife in a close embrace one morning. With my right hand I was touching her skin, which felt warm and soft, and in contrast I experienced my hand as stiff, wooden, and lifeless. All of a sudden it came into my consciousness: "You are not touching your woman with your heart." That's why my hand felt so dull. When I thought about why this was so, I realized I felt trapped in my old pattern of not getting enough. The root of this pattern is not love, openness, and trust, which explains why my hand did not feel loving, trusting, and open. I decided to watch my hand as I shifted my attention away from the pattern to a deep and relaxed presence toward myself. Very swiftly my sensation of my hand changed. My hand softened, became alive, and was gently tingling. Immediately the breath was flowing through my hand and became one with my whole body. My hand was reconnected, and I was again able to touch from the heart. I was aware of the whole and no longer focused on my pattern. This experience taught me what is most important when touching my wife: relaxed, loving presence toward myself. So every touch is a delight and a touch of my heart.

Tantric Inspiration

If you can go on growing in this intimacy, which is no more excitement, then the joy will arise: first excitement, then love, then joy. Joy is the ultimate product, the fulfillment. Excitement is just a beginning, a triggering; it is not the end. And those who finish at excitement will never know what love is, will never know the mystery of love, will never know the joy of love. They will know sensations, excitement, passionate fever, but they will never know the grace that is love. They will never know how beautiful it is to be with a person with no excitement but with silence, with no words, with no effort to do anything. Just being together, sharing one space, one being, sharing each other, not thinking of what to do, what to say, where to go, how to enjoy; all those things are gone. The storm is over and there is silence.

And it is not that you will not make love but it will not be a making really; it will be a love happening. It will happen out of grace, out of silence, out of rhythm; it will arise from your depths, it will not be bodily really. There is a sex which is spiritual, which has nothing to do with the body. Although the body partakes in it, participates in it, it is not the source of it. Then sex takes on the color of Tantra, only then.

OSHO, TRANSCRIBED TEACHINGS,
LET GO!: A DARSHAN DIARY

7

DATES, FOREPLAY, KISSING, AND POSITIONS

MAKE LOVE DATES

Knowing you are going to have sex can really be a big turn-on. Nothing beats looking at your diary and seeing that from 6 to 9 p.m. tonight you have an appointment with your partner—to make love! You know that *today*, for sure, it's going to happen, which is not generally guaranteed under ordinary circumstances. How many times does your woman brush you aside before she lets you be close? Several years ago there was a story about the famous musician, Sting, and although we don't know whether or not it's true, it makes the point about women's general lack of availability in a humorous way. According to the story, Sting made a comment to the press about his sex life, making himself almost as famous for this as for his music. His claim that he had made love for six hours or so caused an international stir. Some weeks later, or so the story goes, he clarified his statement by explaining that five of the six hours had consisted of begging.

Initially, setting a fixed time for sex may seem somewhat strange, because we have the idea that sex ought to be spontaneous—without preparation or premeditation. In fact, sex is rarely truly spontaneous, but happens more on an accidental or habitual basis. Sexual thoughts accompany man throughout his every day, but although he makes endless appointments for other things, no time or space is consciously set aside for the actual act of sex. Real sex (as opposed to virtual sex, which is increasing at an alarming rate since the advent of the Internet) appears to be low on a man's list of priorities. After work, socializing, putting the kids to bed, and watching TV, then perhaps (if he's not too tired) sex will happen. Hopefully, but not necessarily.

Attunement and Relaxation

With guaranteed sex on the horizon, you will perhaps observe yourself feeling more positive, present, and enthusiastic about being alive. You'll feel more at ease knowing that sex will happen, that your partner has actually agreed to meet you and make love. The knowing allows you to settle into yourself in advance, bringing awareness to your body, your legs, perineum, and breath. Inwardly preparing for sex is an effective form of foreplay.

Set aside three or more hours for lovemaking, if possible. It probably sounds like a lot right now, but after a bit of experimentation, three hours may turn out to be a bit on the short side. If three-hour slots are difficult to carve out for yourselves, then settle for one or two hours. Sometimes give yourself an entire day in bed, with breaks for meals and so on. When lovemaking transpires several times on the same day, bodily ease deepens to the extent that bodies enter a state of spontaneous letting-go, undulating, moving, and dancing of their own accord in a divine choreography. In states such as these, the bodies are unable to stop, so you find yourself making love for hours, totally absorbed, present to each split second, unaware of the passage of time.

The Tantric Quickie

The tantric quickie is also highly recommended. Soft penetration for ten, fifteen, or twenty minutes is a perfect way to start off the day. It brings you back home to yourself before you leave home and allows you to relax into the center of your being, which transforms the quality of the day ahead. Last thing at night is also perfect for a tantric quickie, or during an afternoon nap on the weekend. Soft union without erection is so simple and easy; just slip it in, no big performance needed, no great expenditure of energy. You just connect the genitals, relax into the moment, and become present in your body.

Quite possibly the experience of jumping into sex at a fixed time every day feels clinical and unromantic. Also, putting the unerect penis into the vagina (as described in chapter 6) may feel somewhat cold-blooded and technical. You may even feel shy and self-conscious because you are used to making love in the dark or being more concealed. Don't give concerns such as these too much attention, because first impressions fade quickly. Conscious meetings in broad daylight where everything is natural and out in the open are a dream come true for many of us. How easy is this? How sane and sensible is this? Both people are present, willing, and committed. It is ordinary, yet extraordinary. Any initial feelings of awkwardness will soon be replaced by the joy of simplicity and ordinariness, in which you can connect with yourself and your partner in a relaxed and relaxing way.

FOREPLAY

The majority of women, when pressed, will admit that the usual ways men touch and stimulate them actually turn them off. This is sobering news, but relaxing, too, because it means there is less fumbling and guesswork required. A perfect guideline for foreplay: "It's not *what* you do, but *how* you do it."

Presence and Awareness, the Greatest Aphrodisiac

Osho says, "Tantra denies nothing, but transforms everything," which means that awareness changes the situation; any action carried out with awareness is transformed through awareness itself. This basically means that almost anything goes when we are aware, consenting parties. Best is to keep everything simple, innocent, and exploratory, not following any program or putting yourselves under any pressure. Get into your body and enjoy being in it. Touch, stroke, kiss, embrace, and stay in the awareness. Stay present in each and every movement or gesture, with nowhere special to go, being innocent in the simplicity of the situation.

Any kind of touch should bring about an expansion of the other person's energy field, not a contraction. Foreplay becomes simple with the realization that there is no need to excite your partner to make her horny. Excitement will often cause a contraction of the energy field, and any hard or pressuring physical touch will do the same. Try feather-light touches instead.

What women respond to is man's presence and awareness, and awareness is basically effortless when compared to all the usual action in sex. Of course it initially takes effort to maintain presence, but it becomes increasingly familiar and effortless with practice. Presence is easily accessed through the body, and it takes time for an individual to relax into a cellular experience of self, which naturally captures or holds one in the present.

Patience

Foreplay is not so significant for men, because the male positive pole is more or less ever ready, but women definitely appreciate being given time to warm up to love. A woman requires space to relax into her body, her senses, and her receptivity. As an equal and opposite force, this prerequisite is a basic need for her, as explained in chapter 4. Patience and a selfless approach will pay off for the man in the long term. Patience is not some kind of obligation, but simply realizing, accepting, and appreciating that woman (whom you wish to enter physically) is different from you and needs time to open internally before the marvelous experience of entering and joining with her can be of any true value.

Barry Long said that for man, "Patience is the beginning of stillness." Stillness is a quieting of the system and the lessening of thoughts, staying present in the body and inwardly "holding the space." It is simply being in the here and now, resting in your body and being, present to woman. It is not turning her on, but opening and accessing her, supporting her to relax and melt into herself, giving her the feeling of being at home and at ease. If the initial pace is easy, relaxed, and slow, lovemaking is more likely to be filled with timeless delight and pleasure.

Losing Your Erection

Waiting for, or being with, a woman as her body opens means that most probably you will lose your initial erection, if you have one. Don't worry if this happens! An erection can easily return in an atmosphere of loving presence and awareness. And if not, who cares? You always have the five-star option of soft entry without erection.

Remember, true erection is a by-product of consciousness, love, and presence. It is a magical electromagnetic response to a unique set of circumstances, as explained in chapter 6, which deals with erection in more detail.

The Role of Women's Breasts in Male Erection

The wisest place to give a woman loving attention is her breasts. Woman experience their deepest orgasmic experiences through melting into their breasts. As mentioned earlier, in chapter 4, breasts are the positive dynamic poles of the female body, from which sexual energy is awakened. After some time of relaxing into her breasts (and being supported by her man), a woman will usually feel an overflow, experience a vibrant response, in her vagina. Woman's body then becomes filled with a deep yearning for penetration, and her body and being give an unconditional "yes." When a woman has a strong inner connection to her breasts, the spontaneous erection response is likely to happen more easily (as described in chapter 6).

Woman needs to feel her own breasts for herself, from within. You cannot do the internal feeling for her, but you can definitely create the situation that helps her to feel into, and sense, her breasts from the inside. You can touch both breasts at the same time if you are in a position that allows for a two-hand hold. Otherwise, touching just one breast is also fine, and the woman may wish to touch her other breast herself.

How to Hold the Breasts

With open hands, cup the breasts while lifting upward from underneath them. Let the hand contact be "porous," not compressing or squashing the sensitive breast tissue. Then take your attention into your hands; relax your hands, arms, and shoulders; and simply be present and melt into your hands and into her breasts. Mold your hands to fit the contours. Send love, light, warmth, energy, and good vibrations through your hands into the woman's breasts.

There is no need to stimulate the nipples directly, especially the favored radio-tuner style. Some women become hypersensitive to direct touch of the nipples. For other women, nipple stimulation raises the level of excitement and sometimes triggers orgasm (for both), so they choose to keep things cool. Talk about what kind of touch or hold feels good and helps your woman gain an inner connection to her breasts. Reaching around her body to hold her breasts while you embrace her from behind (right hand—right breast, left hand—left breast) can be a beautifully opening and healing experience for a woman. Right hand on the left breast, left hand on the right breast is also a possibility, where man's arms cross over in front of woman's body. But be careful when crossing the arms. Doing so can make the embrace too tight, which squashes the woman, effectively compressing her energy field and her capacity for relaxation and expansion. She may want to escape your hold instead.

In the situation where a woman has had surgical removal of her breast or breasts, the deeper energy centers remain unaffected. Women will continue to feel the expansion of energy in the breasts even in the absence of the physical breast.

Basically with women there are no general rules to be made. What works one day may not necessarily work the next day. Women are very sensitive to any signs of male intention. Woman can feel immediately if a man has intention behind his touch, and this very often closes down her body. Drop your agendas and programming when you are with a woman. Just be present in yourself and in your heart, sharing your being, touching, and caressing with love. Finding a touch without intention is a subtle art.

In the past it may have appeared that a woman functions counter to the man, in that she demands this, needs that, and has many preconditions to be satisfied before she opens sexually. But we now realize that the obstacle is due to a misunderstanding about her body, and not some kind of mental resistance, personality difference, or lack of interest in sex. Sadly, during the lifetime of a woman the female sexual energy is not often awakened sufficiently for her to have deep orgasmic experiences.

By beginning with her breasts instead of stimulating her clitoris, you will access a woman's sexual energy on a profound inner level. The more a man is able to simply wait for his woman's sexual temperature to rise, to meet and equal his own sexual temperature, the more satisfying the sexual experience is likely to be. Man's deepest longing is to bring woman to orgasmic fulfillment and feel her love flowing toward him.

Oral Sex and Masturbation

Oral sex and mutual masturbation are given a great deal of emphasis in the conventional style of sex because of their stimulating and exciting effects. When we start to create a more relaxed and sensitive environment, the need for stimulation is reduced. So it is possible that in time some things that you previously enjoyed or gave a value to slip out of significance because they no longer serve you. Many men have told us that they reduced their masturbation habit when they experienced how it was having a desensitizing effect on the tissues of the penis.

You may also find another way to do the same thing, remembering that "tantra denies nothing but transforms everything." Touch yourself or the other with love and awareness. Bring their or your body to life, a state of being awake and alert. Get into your senses and sensuality. Expand the pleasure through relaxation. Explore the valleys long before you think of heading for the peak, or perhaps you don't even bother to go there this time. Experiment with how it feels to retain your vital juices.

TANTRIC KISSING

Learning to kiss tantric style has great value. You begin to really enjoy kissing and become incredibly kissable at the same time. Some women say they experience kissing as more intimate than sexual union.

Anyone can be an excellent kisser. Just relax your lips with your mouth lightly closed, bring your full attention into your lips, and become present in them. Tantric kissing is done with full, sustained lip contact. This means you don't stop; you stay connected. You remain joined at the lips, which are fused in a relaxed, sensual fashion. You get together and stay together, so a tantric lip kiss can easily last a few hours. Each person enters the lips with presence and awareness, becoming their lips.

The tongue is usually not used in tantric-style kissing; or if it is, only a little, and delicately. Perhaps the tip of your tongue gently caresses the lips. The famous French tongue kiss can cause a sharp rise in the level of man's excitement and encourage early ejaculation, which means the tongue ought to be used with caution.

Like most things, kissing takes practice, so do not abandon the tantric kiss before you "get it." Suddenly one day it will click. There is nothing obvious to be seen from the outside (except that you do not stop)—a kiss is a kiss—but from within, the experience can be electrifying.

POSITIONS DURING SEX

Positions are relatively unimportant. One position is as good as the next if you enjoy it and it works for you. What is most important is to be present in a position and for the position to enhance the correspondence of penis and vagina, so that it encourages and supports the flow of life force. In general, the actual physical fitting together is maintained as much as possible in any given situation.

Changing Positions through Rotating Moves

Changing position increases awareness and enhances presence. Positions can be changed regularly in order to renew and refresh the environment of the penis and vagina. Positions can be changed when there is a need to move, the pull to sleep, or the urge to stretch.

The sequences of what we call rotating positions are shown in figures 7.1 and 7.2. These are changes of position using circular, dimensional movements, rotating around a focal point—penis inside the vagina. As the bodies move, they endeavor to maintain the connection between penis and vagina. If the penis slips out, just quickly slip it in again. Man can do it, woman can do it—whatever is easiest. Nothing is lost if this happens, but a sense of humor helps.

The starting point of the sequences in figures 7.1 and 7.2 is the scissors position used for soft penetration as described in chapter 6. Scissors is a good beginning position—man on his side, woman on her back, relaxed and easy for both. Scissors position is equally wonderful for slow penetration with erection and is a comfortable position for a short sleep.

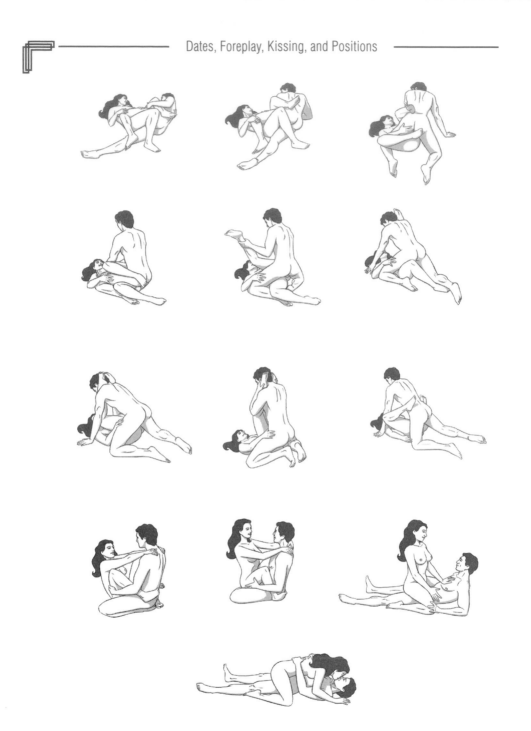

Fig. 7.1. Sequence of rotating positions through front approach

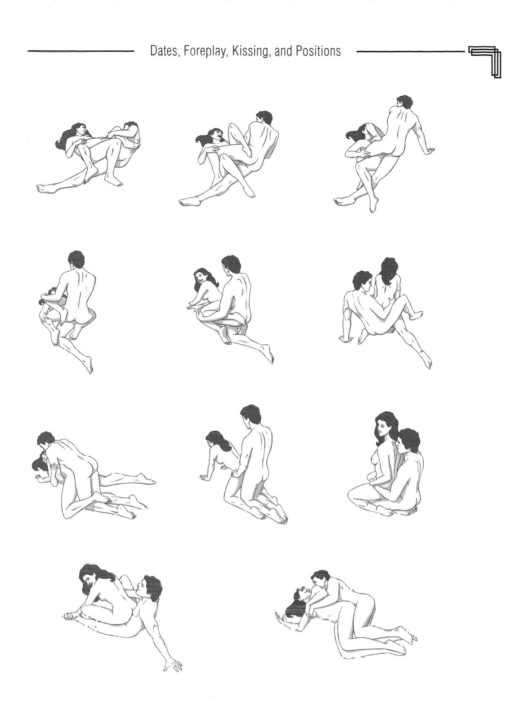

Fig. 7.2. Sequence of rotating positions through rear approach

After five, fifteen, or fifty minutes the position can be changed, as often as necessary, as often as desired. Shifts in position can be done slowly, all movements in a deliberate, step-by-step, unhurried, unfolding and rearranging of bodies.

Tantric Inspiration

And while making love, forget about orgasm. Rather, be in a relaxed state, relax into each other. The Western mind is continuously thinking about when it is coming and how to make it fast and great and this and that. The thinking does not allow the body energies to function. It does not allow the body to have its own way; the mind goes on interfering . . .

Relax . . . If nothing happens there is no need for anything to happen. If nothing happens then that is what is happening . . . and that too is beautiful! Orgasm is not such a thing that it has to happen every day. Sex should be just being together, just dissolving into each other. Then one can keep making love for half an hour, for one hour, just relaxing into each other. Then you will be of utter mindlessness, because there is no need for the mind. Love is the only thing where the mind is not needed; and that is where the West is wrong: it brings in the mind even there.

OSHO, TRANSCRIBED TEACHINGS,
THE OPEN SECRET

PERSONAL SHARING
Finally Getting Enough

My biggest source of stress has been not getting enough sex. Two factors have helped to considerably diminishing this source of stress. First: I have learned to plan sex. Planned sex! Only a short time ago this would have sounded terrible to me. I thought sex had to be spontaneous, there had to be butterflies in the stomach, and I had to be horny, otherwise it wouldn't work. This has changed totally. Nowadays I am planning sex with my wife. On Mondays at 8 p.m., for at least an hour or two, we make time for love. Week by week we have a second look as to when we want to schedule time for sex. This doesn't eliminate spontaneity. Spontaneous love encounters often happen when we're on vacation, but during the normal workweek, it happens rather seldom. With this schedule we make time for something that is very important for both of us. For me this is a great relaxation from the tension of not getting enough. I know that at least once, and maybe twice, per week I will have sex. Wonderful, isn't it? The reason planned sex is nearly always possible is because of tantra. I learned to meet my wife without focusing on sexual desire and excitement. Nowadays I seldom use the word sex; I talk about making love. When we make love, we first tune in, in the form of a common meditation. Each time it is a treat to encounter myself, to open up, to go into my own male power before engaging with my wife. For some time we had put aside meditation preceding lovemaking. Then we often got caught up in discussions, the energy didn't flow, or just about nothing else happened. Generally the lovemaking gets easier, more loving, and more intense if I meditate beforehand.

Secondly. Through tantra, our love is lifted into a totally new dimension. It is fulfilling, sustaining, and very alive. The knack is (and this is really true) to be aware of myself during the lovemaking. This is the opposite of my previous belief that I should do anything possible to make the sex act enjoyable for my wife, and my expectation that she would lead me to a great orgasm as soon as possible.

Tantric Inspiration

In meditation, if two meditators share their energies, love is a constant phenomenon. It does not change. It takes on the quality of eternity. It becomes divine. The meeting of love and meditation is the greatest experience in life, and only then does duality between man and woman disappear.

OSHO, TRANSCRIBED TEACHINGS,
THE REBELLIOUS SPIRIT

8

SEXUAL HEALING AND MALE AUTHORITY

Every fifth woman a man meets in the Western world is likely to have been sexually abused, according to official statistics, and this number does not include women who prefer not to disclose their histories. Perhaps we can even say that every woman has been inadvertently abused or misused to a certain extent, due to the relatively aggressive and hard (unconscious) conventional style of sex. Culturally there is deep misunderstanding about the female body and the way it opens and responds to male energy (see chapter 4). Likewise, because of lack of awareness and information, the way men generally use their bodies in sex is actually abusive to their intrinsic male energy and creates a kind of "overcharge" or disturbance in their systems.

Many men feel a heartfelt concern and unease about the pain and suffering women have been subjected to through sex. At the same time, men feel quite helpless and powerless, and unable to extend support or healing to women on such a sensitive level. Sexual abuse has long-lasting, injurious effects on the life of a woman. The memories in her body and the scars in her psyche can fundamentally affect her capacity to love and enjoy her body and sex. At times in a relationship, abuse issues from the past can reappear out of the blue, become reactivated in the present, and turn into a source of conflict and unhappiness. A man may even carry a lurking guilt about sex in general, in view of the sexual injustices a woman may have experienced in her past. Following the guidelines below will give man a positive alternative and direction for his energy, which is just as beneficial and healing for him as it is for a woman.

This chapter is dedicated to sexual healing and male authority and completes the generative or meditative sexual orientation that we give our retreat participants toward the end of the weeklong retreat. A few threads from themes of earlier chapters will be picked up and drawn together here into a single frame. There will be glancing references to aspects previously addressed in more detail.

VAGINA, NOT CLITORIS

Here we will explain in concrete terms how to deepen our sensitivity so that man and woman become more sensitized in relation to each other. We first need to examine the role of the clitoris and how this has affected woman's capacity to receive. In conventional sex, the clitoris is generally considered by both women and men to be central to female sexuality and orgasm. This leads to a tendency to focus on the clitoral area, which actually lies well outside of the vagina. In addition, within the first few inches of the vagina are some muscular rings that constrict the penis, stimulating it slightly with pleasurable sensations. Because of these considerations, the movement of the penis usually consists of short, repeated, frictionlike thrusts that enter only the first part of the vagina.

These two factors have also caused an external focus in woman, so that her awareness is drawn downward, toward the front of the vaginal/

clitoral area, and away from the deeper regions of the vagina, where, in fact, she is most receptive. Often during hard sex women deliberately have to contract the vagina to close and protect the sensitive cervix (as mentioned before) because it can be painful. Sometimes the deeper area will also contract and "close down" due to the tension of old memories buried deep in the vaginal tissues. These stored memories might include overstepped boundaries, aggressive sex, abusive sex, rape, abortion, gynecological visits, or even anxiety learned from parents or church.

Female Receptivity and Stored Tension

Anxiety, memories, and the external focus on the clitoris result in the deeper regions of the vagina moving out of woman's awareness and thereby becoming a bit inaccessible. There will usually be a corresponding lack of awareness and vitality higher in the vagina. At the same time, most women recognize the significance of this deeper place in their bodies and would like their man to stay deep within what we call the "garden of love" that lies at the entrance to the uterus—the cervix. Even if a woman has had her garden of love area (or the entire uterus) surgically removed for medical reasons, the energy center remains intact and will continue to be a place where woman longs to be touched. But in the normal course of events, man usually reverses out again before woman has a chance to say a word. The place where she is most receptive, most feminine, and best able to experience divine feminine nectar is not available to her, and thereby not available to her man. When an area is closed down there is a lack of inner perception or sensitivity, which can affect a woman's receptivity and sexual experience.

For example, if a woman has a history of sexual abuse, therapy can help to release the trauma, but memory fragments usually remain stored on a cellular level in the tissues, disturbing female receptivity. Fortunately, by the grace of nature, we have been given one magical instrument that can remove these memories and tensions from a woman and awaken her receptivity and femininity—the penis. There are other methods of internal vaginal massage that release tensions by using a finger. However, compared to the magnetic, silky head of the penis, the tip of the finger is almost as rough and crude as sandpaper. Further, there is no real energetic connection between fingers and vagina when compared to the inherent electromagnetic potential between penis and vagina.

THE PENIS AS HEALING CATALYST

The head of the penis is like a highly sensitive magnet with the capacity to draw out disturbing tension. It purifies vaginal tissues, purifying itself in the process, so that there is a reciprocal cycle of purification. Men have their own accumulated traumas and memories from the way we have used and abused our penises. And many men have also been victims of childhood sexual abuse, and carry memories and tensions relating to the experience.

It's important to realize that the penis is not like a vacuum cleaner that sucks up all the woman's tension, leaving you stuck with a full bag. It is more like a catalyst that precipitates the release of tension. The penis causes tension to be released from the system. Through this process man's tensions soften, his male energy gets refined, and the penis loses its overcharge and becomes more supple, pliable, sensitive, and relaxed.

This is very good news, because while an unconscious penis can cause a lot of damage, a conscious penis can create tremendous healing. One of the reasons why the world is suffering from so much war and so many natural disasters is that male and female forces are out of balance. Over the centuries woman (and the feminine energy) has not been treated at all nicely, and while it's perhaps less obvious in Western society, the way woman is still treated today in some cultures is shocking. Man has used and abused woman for his own selfish reasons and when she was no longer interesting, thrown her away and taken another woman. Frequently woman is also used by man to discharge his inner tensions and emotions (see chapter 9). Even if this is not your personal history as a man, the collective human memories over centuries are probably stored in every woman.

Conscious Love Can Heal the Past

By entering woman consciously, in love and presence, man can have an impact on the larger planetary imbalance. It's as if woman is burdened with this collective past that she cannot shake off, but which can be "displaced" and released by a conscious, loving penis—freeing woman and bringing her back to her essential self, which is love. And in purifying woman of her tensions, man is also purified. There is an innate circle of reciprocity; man heals and balances woman, who in turn heals and balances man. By welcoming man in at this level, woman brings him into a state of purity, relaxation, and love (as opposed to fostering the insecure, defensive, and aggressive stance that leads to war). Nature is truly remarkable.

There is a beautiful talk by Barry Long called "Love Brings All to Life," in which he recounts the Greek myth of Pygmalion (see Recommended Books and Resources). Pygmalion was a sculptor who carved a life-sized statue of what he considered to be the perfect woman—the woman of his dreams. He worked passionately, and when he was finally finished, he fell in love with her. He caressed and admired his idealized woman in stone with so much tenderness, so much love and longing that the statue came to life.

Long perceived contemporary women as being in a similar situation. Woman comes into this world already a bit hard, a bit stoney and protective, and for very good reason. She has been abused and misused for much too long, so she is often born with defenses and not truly open to love. Long said that like Pygmalion, man must use the power of his love to soften and melt woman so that she can give up her hardness and protection and return to being pure love.

Female versus Male Essence

Woman in her essence is pure, unconditional love. Man in his essence is pure presence, pure meditation. There are two ways, or polarities, on the spiritual path: one is of love and devotion, and the other is of meditation, presence, and being here now. Osho says these are the two highest polarities in existence; love is female, and presence is male. As woman relaxes in love, meditation or presence grows by itself. As man relaxes into meditation and being present, unconditional and pure love grows by itself.

Through cellular purification woman can once again experience her birthright as pure love. Likewise, man learns to relax into his essence rooted in the present and, very specifically, present in woman in his penis. This is what a woman most wants from a man, that he be present to her. She is not so interested in a great performance as a lover, but that man be present to her while he is inside her. Some men may question this, because often women ask for hard and aggressive sex, but this is more a reflection of her sexual conditioning whereby she has become slightly male herself. It is up to woman to examine this response pattern in herself.

STAYING PRESENT

The capacity to be present really defines what it means to be a man, particularly in light of our cultural confusion. Men are looking for some kind of male authority, but what does it actually mean to be a man? It is nothing less or more than the capacity to be present.

If man can be present in woman—not enter her with a hungry or demanding penis (an emotional penis, see chapter 9), but with a penis that is loving in the here and now—then the penis can begin to "catalyze" what has accumulated in the female body and allow her to relax and transform into pure love—the true quality of woman. For a man there is nothing more gratifying than to see transformation happening before your eyes. Far from being a burden or a job, it feels more like a noble task, an honor to be in woman in a conscious way. To be a chosen one. It gives me (Michael) a certain trust in myself—a male authority. Many men confide at the end of the retreat that they finally have a constructive vision of manhood, and that it is a life-changing experience. And yes, when you cooperate with your sexual nature you do mature and emerge as more of a man. You are more present, relaxed, and connected to your being; you are a more loving human being.

Altering History

Man can do tremendous damage to woman because she represents the container, the space, the environment. Man can leave all his tensions there for selfish reasons, but by putting himself in a larger frame of mind, he actually has the power to change the course of history. That which has been out of balance for thousands of years can start to change today.

There are no mass solutions for the world's problems. There is only one solution, and it starts with this man and this woman. If you can bring the balance back, here in this couple create harmony between man and woman, you do true peace work for the world. And really, there is no other way. You will see that when balance is created here, in the relationship, it radiates out to the world in a palpable way. So some-times perhaps we feel, "Oh, this is boring . . . not so exciting." Always put yourself into a bigger frame of mind, remembering that we are con-nected to a much greater energy field encompassing all of us.

DEEP, SUSTAINED PENETRATION

How do we go about deepening polarity, purification, and healing on a practical level? When erection is present you enter the vagina very slowly (see chapter 6), and you look for places that feel painful, strange, weird, or numb—and you stay exactly on that spot. Sensitive, painful spots can be anywhere—just inside the entrance of the vagina, along the walls, or in the upper regions, the "garden of love." Woman will help you to identify these places. We suggest you maintain soft eye contact as described in chapter 7. Open eyes help to keep you present and avail-able, and subtle reactions and responses expressed in her eyes can some-times give you information about what is happening internally.

Usually pain is something we avoid; we do not like to touch sensi-tive areas, naturally, because doing so is painful. But now we are inten-tionally looking for them. Pain or lack of sensitivity (deadness) indicates held tension and memories in the vaginal tissues. By going in there very consciously, with great awareness, it's possible to contact these areas with the penis. Woman will usually allow this because you do not push into the pain, you just want to gently contact the pain. You make a "porous" contact with the area. You don't want to push hard against the vaginal walls, because that would reinforce woman's protective instinct. You find a sensitive area, and then you pull back a hairsbreadth—more like a withdrawal of intention. This creates space for an interaction of ener-gies, so that things can shift. You just stay there without moving; you sustain the contact in the depths. Your woman can use simple words to communicate what is happening, and you can do the same. This begins a journey of discovery over a period of time, touching all sides of the vagina, the entire canal, seeking out those areas we usually avoid.

If a woman has pain at the very entrance of the vagina, you can just place the head of your penis there and let it rest. Often penetration becomes very painful when women go through menopause, and this approach relaxes the tension. If the movement of the penis in the vagina has a burning sensation for a woman, it can mean that the entry is too fast. Ask your woman if she feels any burning. If she does, stop, withdraw half an inch or so, and wait for a little while to enable the vaginal tissues to soften and relax. Then move again, very slowly, and stop as soon as your woman again reports burning sensations. At times an additional, generous application of oil to the head of the penis and to the vaginal lips and opening will counteract any burning sensations.

Some women experience painful penetration throughout their sexual lives. Recently a woman in our group had a pain-free penetration for the very first time in her life, after forty years of every sexual experience being painful. Just the head of the penis can do so much healing, so try this healing approach any time you wish. Let it be a new orientation. Pain is interesting; it is a doorway, and there is usually treasure hidden behind that pain.

Loss of Erection

When you find painful areas and stay in contact with them, you might suddenly start to lose your erection. Usually when this happens we will try to get the erection back as fast as possible, but now in this new situation we understand that this is the way the penis does the job. When the penis has done its job, it is going to be relaxed, naturally. Like everything in life, there is an active phase and a passive phase, but in sex we want an active erection all the time, 100 percent.

If you accept this relaxation of the penis from time to time and do not interfere with its withdrawal, you allow your penis the opportunity to regenerate. Often, just as the penis is about to slip out of the vagina entirely, it will again begin reaching out, spiraling upward and erecting in the vagina (see chapter 6). Soon you may get the feeling that the genitals themselves are making love and that actually they know how to do it better. It is almost like handing the intelligence back to the body, and it is such a remarkable experience that you can almost lean back and watch the show.

Trust Your Penis

The experience of my penis responding of its own accord gives me a trust in myself, because basically we men do not trust our penises; they are not completely reliable. But when I know that this is going to be the process, then I can trust my penis, and that gives me trust in myself as a man. I no longer feel I need to be strong or ambitious, need to prove this and that. My definition of man has changed. The only thing that is required from me, as man, is to be present, to develop the capacity to be here now. Then miracles are possible.

When there is erection, you enter as far as you can go and sustain the penetration; you stay where you are. We call this deepening polarity through deep, sustained penetration, because as the woman gets more receptive, man gets more dynamic, and the potential between male and female poles increases. In general in your life, as a style of lovemaking, you begin to "hang out" deep in the vagina, allowing the dynamic and receptive forces to start to play with each other. Here woman is "minus" while man is "plus," and any obstructions (tensions) lying in the way of this moving magnetic force are displaced so that healing, purification, and regeneration can take place.

The effects of deep, sustained penetration also work with and through condoms; the energy exchange is relatively unaffected (see more about condoms in chapter 6).

Effectiveness and Penis Length

Some men worry that the penis may not be long enough to reach all the way up to the "garden of love." Both women and men have reported to us that the cervix also seems to be drawn downward as it reaches for the head of the penis. Always remind yourself that these are energetic phenomena, not purely physical, and the energy exchange works in any case. Even with a soft, relaxed penis that remains still within the first couple of inches of the vagina, purification and healing is taking place.

Unexpected Ejaculation

During deep, sustained penetration, at times a woman's buried tensions are suddenly discharged down the vagina, almost like a rush or wave of excitement. This can easily cause a man to ejaculate instantly, without any warning. Should it happen, do not feel something went wrong—it's a natural part of the purification process.

ALLOW OLD FEELINGS TO SURFACE

As you make love and pay attention to places in the vagina that are painful or numb, it is likely that for your partner tears, sadness, or anger may come to the surface. You yourself might experience similar feelings. This is all good. These feelings are trapped and held in the body, and the old must come out to create space for the new. Expressing previously unexpressed feelings (see chapter 9) cleanses our poles, our genitals, and our bodies become more sensitive and sensitized. One becomes increasingly receptive, the other increasingly dynamic.

Don't try to figure out what's happening when old, buried feelings or emotions emerge. Thinking about what is going on distances you from the experience, so just stay with the feelings and allow them to flow. Sometimes spontaneous understanding will occur, an insight into the source of the pain, but not necessarily. Healing takes place in any event.

If uncomfortable feelings start to arise, be aware that it is not the fault of your partner. Your partner is simply a trigger to help you to retrieve the past. Old feelings stored in the cells are going to rise to the surface, offering the opportunity to finally express feelings you may have been storing since childhood. So if suddenly a lot of tears come up, don't think, "Oh, now I have to be alone to deal with my old feelings" (see "golden rules" in chapter 9). No, it is the genital connection that is triggering the release of old feelings, so just stay together inside each other. Or if suddenly anger pops up, which can easily happen, you can simply explain, "I'm just really angry, I have to move this energy." Then you disconnect and quickly do something physical, like jumping up and down, to burn up the anger. As soon as you feel the wave of anger has passed, climb back into bed and continue making love. Through a polarity exchange, purification is happening on both sides, and it changes your whole experience and sense of yourselves as man and woman.

Self-healing

We talk more frequently about the abuse of women, because they do suffer more abuse, but many men, too, are carrying a history of pain, insecurity, and self- or other-inflicted abuse in their bodies, so it is important to understand that sexual healing is not only for woman. It really is a self-healing that happens through awareness and channeling and directing energy in a constructive way. After a time any pains will usually disappear.

Sometimes you might lie in bed and just cry and cry, perhaps not only for yourself, but for all of humanity. If you allow yourself to be washed through, you will experience how much it empowers you to feel the pain of humanity flowing through you. So avoid trying to understand what's going on; just accept it with gratitude.

When we first met we spent days and days, three weeks crying. I (Michael) don't know what or why, except that it was just wonderful. It felt like very old pain, and at the same time was exquisitely beautiful.

Communicate, Share, Express

As you make love in this way you communicate all of what's happening—strange feelings, numbness, beautiful sensations—in simple words. Do not try to explain anything; just acknowledging is enough. Sometimes when tension is released there is laughter. So whether it is tears, laughter, shivering, shaking, or sweating, simply allow it and be with it. These are all signs of the body purifying and detoxifying the cells of past memories.

POSITIONS SUITABLE FOR DEEP, SUSTAINED PENETRATION

Since the painful places can be anywhere in the entire vagina and cervix area, there is quite a lot of room to explore, and many angles can be used. A variety of positions are suitable, as suggested in the diagrams (see figures 8.1–8.7). However, even subtle shifts of the penis in the vagina, moving one centimeter and staying there, represent a shift in position. You do not have to always move your entire body, but instead reach to different parts of the vagina through subtle shifts in the angle of the pelvis. Positions are covered in more depth in chapter 7, where the basic guideline is that positions per se are not as significant as the level of awareness that a person brings to them. Any position is perfect when it feels right.

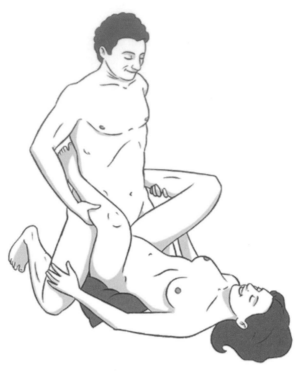

Fig. 8.1. Middle position, man kneeling
(with pillow to raise woman's pelvis)

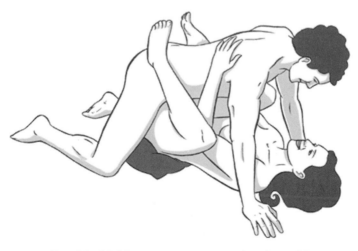

Fig. 8.2. Middle position, man on hands and knees
(with pillow to raise woman's pelvis)

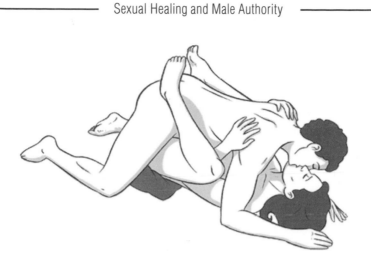

Fig. 8.3. Middle position, man lying forward, half kneeling
(with pillow to raise woman's pelvis)

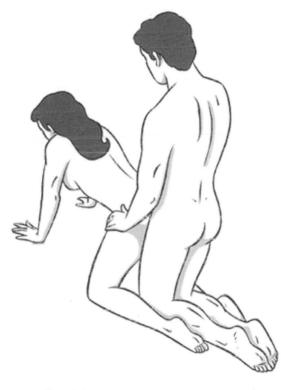

Fig. 8.4. Rear position with man kneeling

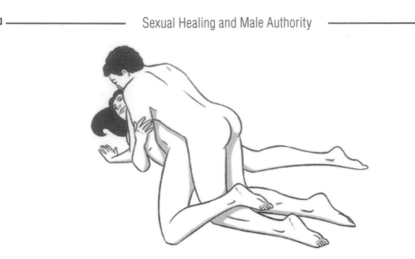

Fig. 8.5. Rear position with man lying on top of woman

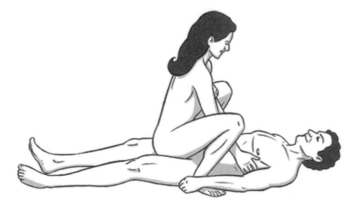

Fig. 8.6. Woman sitting on top

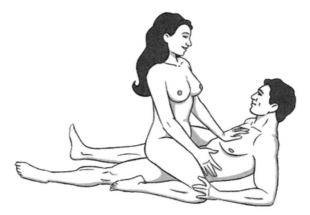

Fig. 8.7. Woman kneeling on top

PARTNERING WITH WOMEN

If woman has the garden of love, then we men are the "gardeners of love." We have to take care, remove the weeds, and plant roses. When man becomes rooted in his penis as a positive force, he experiences true male authority with the capacity to heal woman of her past. Sex can be lived as a spiritual, loving meditative force, becoming the roots of powerful self-healing and transformation.

On the surface it may appear as if man has to tune into woman and do it her way, or that tantra is for women and not for men, but the issue extends to deeper levels. In making love from the inner dimension, man will discover his true male authority. He will certainly feel a new authority or competence when he is able to open the heart of woman with his penis. Allowing woman to be the guide may be unexpectedly fulfilling. Yes, after thousands of years it does seem intelligent to make a change, and to realize that it is for male empowerment in the long term. If we want to have more love in our lives, make love to women, and have women want to make love to us, we have to allow women to help us to find our true inner man.

Easy, Natural Orgasms

Often woman say, "I don't really feel that I lose energy with the conventional orgasm. How does this fit into the picture?" The approach to take regarding orgasm is not to take an approach. You don't want to go looking for orgasm, hunting or pushing for it. But when an orgasm happens easily and naturally, with no effort, then it is beautiful. So first a woman really has to observe and ask herself, "Am I relaxing into the moment or am I pursuing—even a little bit—orgasm?" In general, if woman allows the clitoris to be more passive and fade into the background, she will find it easier to take her awareness higher up into the vagina where her divine energies are accessed.

Woman's Healing Contribution

Basically women, as the receptive element, are very vulnerable; their one and only defense is to deny man entry. Women's no to sex can be a reflection of a painful personal or collective history, but in either case it's a by-product of our cultural lack of sexual information. So what a woman can do for this healing process is to start to say yes to man when he is committed to being conscious inside her. Woman can begin to allow him in so that healing can begin. She can step beyond sexual politics and invite the male force inside of her. Through this a tremendous amount of healing is possible for both woman and man.

Over the centuries sex and love have become two separate things entirely. Much too often sex has nothing to do with love, but when a woman allows man to enter and be present in her in consciousness, aspects that have been separated for centuries can reunite. Sex (the lower vibration) and love (the higher vibration) of the same life force become one expression. When we understand how bodies cooperate, we can completely change our inherited sexual patterns.

PERSONAL SHARING
The Joy of Feeling Welcome

Tantra helps me to tap in to the unexplored aspects of my being. Even without pursuing the goal of becoming more conscious of deep-rooted patterns, primal fears come up from time to time while practicing tantra. And at the same time, it leads me into dimensions, takes me toward energies I would not have reached and felt without tantra and without my wife. The following situation brings up the most significant sensations: Whenever my penis is softly lying in the vagina of my wife, its mere presence creates a deep connection between the male and the female pole. I have the sense that I am pulled in by her vagina, yet I also feel that by my penis stiffening, my male energy is growing into my woman. The sensation of being pulled in to her vagina is one of the most beautiful feelings that I know. It tells me on a very deep level: "You are welcome." One of my deepest fears is that I might not be welcome, so to experience this welcome again and again relaxes me in the depths of my soul. This fear is a basic fear of all manhood. Many men have confirmed this by sharing with me that they personally have this primal fear. When I first had this experience of being pulled in to a woman (during the tantra course) I was simply overwhelmed. I had never expected to experience being so deeply welcomed, ever in my life. I just cried with joy, but also because such a deep pain started to be released. Today I can honestly say that the fear of not being welcome, not getting enough and being rejected, has largely been healed.

PERSONAL SHARING
Penis Tension Resolved

Besides the changes on the spiritual-energetic level, I also feel changes on the physical plane. Previously, when I touched the top of my penis, the sensation was always partly unpleasant. It made me back off inside and become tense. I experienced that as a defensive tension in the tissue. As far as I can remember, it had always been like that. Four months after the tantra course, this unpleasant part dissolved and has not returned. I am surprised by this experience, but it teaches me that my body becomes soft, vulnerable, and receptive through tantra.

The most important experience with tantra is that each time it is different; nothing happens twice in the exact same way. It's like life itself — every day brings something new. Therefore, I experience tantra as a precious teacher for my whole life.

Tantric Inspiration

What is love? Love is the fragrance, the radiance of knowing oneself, of being oneself. . . . Love is overflowing joy. Love is when you have seen who you are; and then there is nothing left except to share your being with others. Love is when you have seen that you are not separate from existence. Love is when you have felt an organic orgasmic unity with all that is. Love is not a relationship. Love is a state of being. It has nothing to do with anybody else. One is not in love; one is love. And of course, when one is love, one is in love—but that is an outcome, a by-product, that is not the source. The source is that one is love.

OSHO, TRANSCRIBED TEACHINGS,
THE GUEST

9
MASTERING LOVE AND OVERCOMING EMOTIONS

Tantra sees human energy in terms of polarity: feminine energy as "being" and masculine energy as "doing." Within woman, the inner masculine is active, logical, and result oriented; and in man, the inner feminine is receptive, intuitive, and process oriented. Tantra takes a step further to say that the highest spiritual polarity in existence is love and meditation, that woman embodies love and man embodies meditation. This implies that woman's inner man is meditative and man's inner woman is loving.

To be whole human beings, operating with wisdom, passion, authenticity, and spontaneity, we need to master both energies: masculine and feminine, meditation and love. Woman becomes more meditative the more she loves, and man becomes more loving the more he meditates. In more precise sexual language, to love in woman means to welcome the penis in and surrender to its power, and to meditate in man means to merge with, and become fully present in, his penis, inside woman, in stillness.

DISTINGUISHING
BETWEEN EMOTIONS AND FEELINGS

Deep personal and societal wounding prevents many of us from balancing our energies in a way that serves us. We repress the memories of our hurts, suppress our real feelings and energies, and then unconsciously begin to control or manipulate others, or fail to channel our energies in a wise or creative direction. As we change the way we make love, we initiate an alchemical process of awakening the inner, opposite polarity, which will, in time, enable us to use both energies powerfully and productively. This, in turn, helps us to dissolve emotional patterns that have caused us pain in the past and enables us to create the life and love we long for in the present.

To create the life of sustained, loving harmony that so many of us wish for, an important step is to keep emotion out of love. As Osho says, "Love is a state of being," and "One is not in love, one is love . . . it has nothing to do with anybody else." With the new input about harnessing polarity and our orgasmic potential, we might be able to conceive of days of "being love" as a sustained state that is not associated with the highs and lows of relationships. But what about these highs and the painfully difficult, emotion-laden lows, when love becomes scrambled up with irreconcilable feelings and fears? Despair or resignation can set in when a couple can see no way out of the cycle of conflicts.

Regaining our power in love is dependent on knowing the difference between feelings and emotions, knowing that "love has to be separated from this category of emotions." (See the tantric inspiration at the end of this chapter.) It is crucial to understand that emotion comes from the past, while love and true feelings arise in the present. When too much "emotional baggage" from the past gets dragged into everyday life, love is quick to wane; love flourishes in the delicacy of the now. That doesn't mean emotion is some kind of demon. Emotion is understandable, but it's important to be aware that you are emotional and to know what is happening, when it is happening. The recognition of emotionality causes a big shift in the maturity of an individual and a couple.

Symptoms of Emotion

Until now we have had no frame of reference to understand what is truly going on in the split second in which emotions surface—the instant when, seemingly out of the blue, the love boat begins to rock dangerously. What we need is self-awareness. The immediate physical symptoms of emotion can be described variously as "suddenly feeling paralyzed" or as if "a wall suddenly comes down." You may experience a jumble of feelings you can't put into words, find it impossible to look the other in the eyes, or have the awkward sensation of feeling disconnected from everything, utterly separate, lonely, totally misunderstood, and physically collapsed. Often we find ourselves feeling vengeful and wanting to hurt back. We start blaming our partner for the situation, using the accusing words, "You never . . ." or "You always . . ." When a breakdown like this takes place, we must recognize that emotion is in play. It takes some practice to recognize emotion, but after a while, it does become obvious.

This inner acknowledgement immediately puts things into better perspective. Emotion is the resurfacing of old or repressed feelings that we were unable to show or express at the time the feeling was actually taking place. This is why emotional reactions are often quite disproportionate to the slight comment or mild action that triggers them. The trigger itself does not usually warrant the huge upset that follows in its wake. It's those old, unexpressed feelings that begin to resonate and bubble to the surface and create confusion. When you acknowledge these old feelings for what they are and work their negative effects out of your system, emotional reactions will begin to diminish. In a few years your partner will be able to say precisely the same words to you, and the comment will slip by you like water off a duck's back.

The Solar Plexus and Emotion

In addition to emotional alarm signals like suddenly feeling paralyzed or disconnected, you can learn to recognize states of emotionality through your solar plexus. Consider this area as a sensor, because here the tensions of emotions can gather and create a lot of discomfort. These tensions try to seek discharge in various ways—through irritation, complaining, nagging, or passing on your frustration to family members or colleagues. When you develop awareness of the solar plexus, the moment someone says something that strikes an uncomfortable chord in you, you will probably notice a response in that part of your body: the sensation of tension or congestion, like having a stone in your stomach, or a hollow, empty, nervous feeling in the stomach. These kinds of body responses let you know that you are emotional and that something unresolved is being triggered. If the solar plexus is free of tension, it allows for unobstructed flow of sexual energy between the genitals and heart. There may be slight feelings of nausea when first relaxing into lovemaking (perhaps more common in woman), but this is nothing to be concerned about. It is a sure sign of the surfacing of old tensions seeking release. Nausea is usually a by-product of the sexual energy expanding, displacing, and cleansing the restricting tensions from the body.

OVERCOMING FEARS
CREATED BY LACK OF LOVE

Many people begin experiencing feelings of being separate, wrong, unworthy, or not good enough very early in life, already as young children. We become separate from ourselves, from each other, and from the whole of existence. As we cut off from our pure energy, we also cut off from our love source, and as fear replaces security and joy, a false self gradually develops around us. The fear is due to imprints made by an absence of love in the immediate surroundings (family and parents). It provokes a child into behaving differently in order to try to get approval (or disapproval, through rebellion, where at least some attention is gained) and secure the love so necessary for survival. And so our parents begin to write the script for who we are and how we should behave, and we gradually lose our authenticity.

Emotionality is an unconscious, automatic reaction to a situation or circumstance, like when a switch is flicked off, and light turns to dark. It can even be a learned habit: some people learned to be emotional as young children by mimicking their parents' behavior. As the years go by, we begin to define ourselves according to our emotions, thinking our emotional part is who we really are. It is as if we are in a movie, and the situation is not actually real. Only the past makes it real. (If we were to wake up one morning without our memory, with no past, what then?) But in spirit and essence we are all interested in love, and to keep love alive, love has to be separated from the unconscious backlog of stored emotions. As we begin to release these old feelings consciously (whenever we notice them arising), pieces of the past get healed.

Toxic Emotions and Conventional Sex

Emotions are extremely toxic and will poison the atmosphere by striking deadly blows at the person we most love. This is a big problem; we unconsciously put all our unresolved feelings onto the person we most love and thereby contaminate the love. We say the most awful things to our partner in an attempt to unburden ourselves of our emotions. Emotional statements stick like glue in the mind and revolve endlessly in the thoughts, long after the fight is over. Did she really mean that? Am I really like that? And then the mind will create more emotions from endlessly rethinking the past. In truth, love cannot withstand too much emotion; it is a delicate and fragile flower that requires awareness to keep it blooming. Love will slowly slip through our fingers when we let emotion have the upper hand.

A big source of emotionality lies hidden in sex. When energy moves downward, as it does in conventional sex with its usual discharge, tension and anxiety are by-products. This is why arguments and dissatisfactions easily follow. Sexual tensions eventually create a subtle overpositive charge in man and a subtle false-positive charge in woman. These falsely acquired charges make woman slightly male and distort her essential female qualities. Man's essential qualities are also distorted as he becomes a "tough guy." These accumulating tensions have to be discharged in some fashion, and they are often released through arguing, finding fault with each other, or complaining. When emotions are in the air they easily spawn excitement, which gives rise to the famous fucking-after-a-fight syndrome to heal the rift. But trying to repair the damage through sex and ejaculation/orgasm is a vicious cycle, because through that very same fuck we acquire more charge, which can flare up into emotion at any moment. This explains why, even in the absence of an argument, after a so-called good fuck, a fight can start so easily.

Recent brain research has revealed that chemicals released during a conventional peak orgasm have a separating effect that causes withdrawal and disconnection (see Marnia Robinson's book *Cupid's Poisoned Arrow* in Recommended Books). Previously we mentioned a tendency for men and women to withdraw and feel separate after peak orgasms. Now we know that behavior is actually controlled by a chemical event in the brain. Conventional sex ultimately causes separation, not union.

False Female Emotionality

The false charge built up through a misunderstanding about how genitals relate to each other is a big factor in the emotions for which women have become famous. The overcharge, tensions, and stresses present in the system seek release in order to keep the system in some kind of balance. One way they manifest is in the form of overwhelming emotions. Women seem so sensitive, get upset easily and cry, have dramas, and start blaming. This is man's nightmare! These emotional reactions affect a woman's equilibrium and her capacity to love and be loved. The tensions can also be reflected in women as various menstrual syndromes or genital disturbances.

Man unknowingly contributes to this. When man has hot sex and ejaculates, he frequently (but not always) deposits some of his sexual/emotional tension in woman's body, which she later has to process in some way or other. Woman is unconsciously accumulating stress and tension on a few fronts, which affects her behavior and self-perception, and men's perception of women.

The Emotion of Jealousy

Jealousy is perhaps the most debilitating and excruciating of emotions. Jealousy is about having the desire to possess and control another person; it is not an expression of love for that person. Jealousy has its roots in comparison, and we are taught to compare ourselves in all kinds of ways, particularly in the sexual sphere. Comparison is a useless activity because each individual is unique and incomparable, and once you truly understand this, jealousy can evaporate. Sex certainly creates jealousy, but jealousy is a secondary thing, so it is not a question of how to get rid of jealousy. It is more a question of loving without conditions. Love that does not control or posses but honors the other's freedom to live their own life.

GOLDEN RULES FOR
GETTING RID OF EMOTION

There are some "golden rules" (elaborated on in *Tantric Love: Feelings versus Emotions;* see Recommended Books and Resources) to help in processing emotion. The very moment you recognize that you are emotional—through the solar plexus, the experience of disconnection, or in whatever other way you recognize your emotion—the first step is to acknowledge it and say aloud to your partner, "I am emotional." This verbalization instantly brings a touch of relaxation, because at least now your partner knows that you know that you are emotional, which takes the other out of the picture and no longer makes that person responsible for your unhappiness. It is a difficult and challenging step to take (at first), to admit you are emotional by actually saying so, because the ego will be justifying and fighting like crazy, trying to blame the other. But until you take yourself back to yourself and acknowledge the unexpressed past within you, your love life will remain a series of good times followed by bad times.

In such circumstances, having said the three golden words, "I am emotional," to your partner as gracefully as possible, physically leave the room, adding the words, "I need some time to myself and will return soon." Close the door gently and go outside or to another room in the house and take some time alone. (Do not drive off and feign that you are abandoning the relationship in that moment—accidents happen.) Now is not switch-off time, but the time to switch on and release, to get in touch with old feelings residing in your system by moving your body. In fact, when emotions get activated the toxins of feelings gone sour move through a layer of connective tissue in the body, called fascia. This explains why sometimes at the onset of an emotional attack you will feel the event in your body very clearly, almost as if a substance with density is swirling through you. (Indeed, fascia does weave dimensionally through the body and from head to toe about five times, connecting the superficial layers with the deepest physical layers.)

To get rid of these emotions, you need to use physical movement to help them move out of the body. Be active in some way, and do whatever you do purposefully; for example, beat a pillow for twenty minutes, bang on a drum, go for a jog, chop some wood, or dig in the garden. Talking gibberish (nonsensical words) also helps to clear emotion. It's important to be physically active and do what you do with intention and not give in to any inclination to contract and collapse. Surprisingly, when you return to your partner after a bout of physical release you are likely to experience that the feeling of disconnection has diminished, you can make eye contact again, and the distancing "wall" is slowly crumbling to the ground.

If this is not the case, if you feel you are still looking over a half wall, that there's still some sense of separation, you likely need an additional round of body movement. This sounds almost too simple, but it works. If you need two or three hours, or days, to get over the attack of emotion, then take the time required. As you begin to operate in this way with your emotions, soon the whole process gets faster—the recognition, the acknowledgment, and the burning up of the past.

Being creative in this way certainly beats the alternative option of dragging the emotions around for a few days, miserably wondering what has become of love, until eventually, sleepless nights later, one side breaks down into tears, gives up the fight, and starts to express the feelings lurking behind the emotions. You have experienced this yourself many times, for sure; the very instant one side gives up and starts to express inner feelings, the fight is over. We pick up the remaining threads of love and start again.

You may wonder why it is necessary to separate physically in order to deal with emotions. One of the telltale traits of emotion is that it enjoys discussion and argument, each one trying to convince the other why he or she is right. Emotion is full of ego. If you do stay in each other's presence when emotionally activated, it is really best if you can speak only about yourself and say, "I feel . . ." This is the most direct way to step out of emotion, by expressing and releasing your deep, hidden feelings. Bring the congestion of emotions from the solar plexus—where it is likely to have formed a knot—up to the heart, and get into your inner feelings for real. Do not make your partner responsible for creating unhappiness in you. Reach behind the emotion and find what is truly happening inside of you, the old buried hurts that have nothing to do with this individual in front of you. She has only been a trigger.

Even if this person is in some way responsible for some of the hurts you carry from the past, the fact that you repressed your deeper feelings at that time and did not express them is really the issue in the present. If feelings had been authentically released at the time, they would not keep bubbling up inside of you. You would have felt a great deal better for having expressed the feelings, even if a particular issue remained unresolved between you. Through expression you release emotions you've been dragging around and accumulating year by year. You keep yourself free from the past.

THE ROLE OF EMOTIONS IN SEX

Because of our emotional patterns, as couples we tend to get a bit high on emotions and begin to believe that this intensity is a part of love, and that a good hurling of china is an expression of our love. We once heard Barry Long say that all anger is, in reality, the result of sexual frustration. This certainly gives food for thought, especially in light of all the wars going on around us and how little satisfying sex is being enjoyed on Earth. Men and women have pressures and frustrations associated with conventional orgasm, so they are quite likely to have anger about this as well. Many women feel deep rage toward men for their abusive behavior, a rage that extends beyond the personal to the collective level.

Discharging Emotions through Sex

Very often men use sex to discharge their emotional tension. Since they generally express their real feelings much less readily than women, men often have an overload of unexpressed feelings, along with their accompanying tensions. These cause an "itch" in the system, and a man can start to feel horny and want quick sex, excitement, and discharge in order to balance the system. This type of sex has nothing to do with man's basic sexual system and how he is designed to operate as the male principle on Earth. Barry Long referred to the hot excitement/ejaculation style of sex as "emotional sex," and a demanding or hungry or aggressive penis as an "emotional penis."

For man to discover his true male qualities he is advised to refrain from using the sexual channel to release emotional tensions. Ejaculation is certainly an extremely pleasurable way to release them, but there are consequences to such discharges. Men need to find alternative ways to release the tensions they accumulate through life in general, which often involves high levels of stress and anxiety, including survival anxiety. Men will benefit enormously from using their legs in regular daily exercise—for example, jogging, gym workouts, ta'i chi, dance, squats, and any kind of stretching—as well as receiving regular deep-tissue massage in order to relax and free tension in the musculature of the legs and feet.

Tantric Sex Reduces Emotionality

When love is made consciously and emotional or hot sex is avoided (or reduced), there is soon a visible shift in the emotional state of woman. She becomes more radiant, open, and content. Nagging stops, and she begins to flower. Women in our couple's workshops experience a shift within two or three days of making love regularly without forcing a peak orgasm. Men also notice a big change in their own emotional state, as they become calm and centered, grounded in the body, more present and aware, more relaxed, and more loving. Sounds perfect! Men also notice that anger is not provoked so easily. Anger and frustration levels reduce dramatically when hot sex and ejaculation are avoided or reduced.

How we make love profoundly affects who we are and how we conduct ourselves as human beings. It is of eternal value to explore evolved sexual approaches and observe how these experiences begin to shape who you are, how you feel on an inner level, and your perception of each other and the world around you.

EXPRESSING FEELINGS IN THE PRESENT

In addition to keeping the past in the past by recognizing when emotion steps in, and experimenting with relaxing into sex to avoid adding emotions to those you already have, the art now becomes one of staying in touch with your feelings so that you can begin to feel what you are feeling. To keep love fresh and free of emotion it becomes essential to express feelings as they arise. Do not hang on to your feelings for an instant, unless you are in a hopelessly inappropriate situation. Move with the rising feeling and don't let your mind talk you out of it. Allow tears to flow, laughter to erupt, and roars to unleash. Jump up and down, do something fast, and above all, do not repress feelings and in so doing form fresh emotions, which happens very quickly. Equally quickly, any sadness, pain, anger, or frustration, if fully lived as it is happening, will have a life span of about eight intense seconds, after which it is all over.

When you practice consciously expressing anger there are a few hard-and-fast golden rules that come with it, and these are not to be broken under any circumstances. If you feel anger, do not direct it onto your partner, even if your emotions are convincing you that she is at fault. Do not touch her or do anything to hurt her physically; do not even face her. Turn to face in the opposite direction, showing her your back; then let a deep roar emerge from your belly.

PERSONAL SHARING
Releasing the Roar

The first time I consciously allowed my anger to flow was unforgettable. In the very instant that I felt the rising anger for being blamed for something I did not do, I contacted a deep, roaring sound in my belly that was so powerful it shot me up into the air to virtually touch the ceiling, and this one was higher than most ceilings. By the time gravity pulled me back to terra firma a second or two later, it was all over. I felt no anger, no emotion, no resentment—nothing. I stepped back into the moment without hesitation, ready to continue relating, I felt liberated and refreshed.

When anger arises, welcome it, knowing that it is old tension within you that can be transformed. By expressing it you are released from its restrictive grip. Contacting feelings is a cleansing experience; energy that was locked up suddenly becomes available. When you express a feeling or transform an emotion into a feeling you feel lighter, expanded, and fresh; you're more connected to your partner, open and soft, clear and radiant, even loving. Emotions bring the experience of quite opposite qualities: darkness and gloom, despair and collapse. The whole range of positive uplifting experiences arise when you share your feelings. (Learn more in *Nonviolent Communication: A Language of Life*; see Recommended Books and Resources.)

HUMANS NEED LOVEMAKING FOR CONTINUED WELL-BEING

Relaxing into sex brings you into a state of being that is quite apart from the whole range of emotions. Through relaxation we reach a rare state in which our energy is regenerated, and we become suffused with peacefulness as opposed to frustration. As life force moves upward through the energy centers (chakras), it cleanses and purifies them and makes the inner-body experience increasingly dynamic and alive.

Contemporary women suffer from a mass of issues: extreme menstrual syndromes with hormonal ups and downs, poor self-esteem, fears of aging, menopausal anxieties, disappointment, and often disinterest in sex. At a certain point sex is considered by many women to be too much hard work with very little reward, and for this reason they abandon it.

For men the situation is equally dire. Until given the chance to enjoy the expansion of his sexual energy through direct experience, man cannot begin to imagine it. And since excitement and ejaculation are the only experiences he knows, it is not so easy to consider doing something differently. A man's inability to channel his real life force can result in frustration, aggression, anger, restlessness, obsessive fantasizing about sex (both alone and during the act), and all types of sexual perversions.

When the life force circulates freely through man he finally feels himself as more of a man. At the end of a recent workshop a man said, "This is the first time in my life of fifty-four years that I have been given any insight or guidance on what it means to be a man." And that was not the first time we've heard this. When a man knows how to use his sexual energy correctly, allowing it to expand throughout his body, the sense of self changes. Sex becomes less to do with the other or with getting something, and becomes more a way of valuing and loving oneself, of being with oneself. And in this frame woman is likely to be more interested in making love. With insight into our body mechanisms we are able to direct the sexual energy and be more in command of love and life. Man will be in wonder, even a bit awestruck to learn how the same elements—the penis and the vagina—can produce two such vastly different experiences.

MALE AUTHORITY THROUGH TAKING RESPONSIBLE ACTION

Many a man is interested in producing a peak orgasm for a woman because he believes it validates him as a lover, but this attitude has grave consequences for both men and women. Until a man can manage to fully satisfy one woman, he will never feel himself to be a true man, in spite of any other achievements and successes. The need for man to feel himself as masculine, for woman to feel herself as feminine, and for both to have orgasmic experiences through each other is a burning need for humanity today. Without the generative, spiritual, sexual expression, the human race will slowly die from love starvation.

Eliminating or reducing the usual orgasm-driven sex may sound like a loss, but this is truly responsible action on the part of a man. With responsibility you gain freedom, higher sexual experiences, and greater sexual fulfillment, and you transform from an emotional human into a loving human. You lift yourself out of the cycles of unconsciousness that have been going on between people for generations. Life changes its whole quality when the genitals are reserved to serve love, which is their higher purpose. Reproduction is the lower purpose of the sexual interaction. Through understanding the genitals anew and using them according to the inherent polarities embodied in male and female, it is possible to create love in the here and now, with the person you are with today. You learn to contain the energy, embrace it, expand with it, and melt into it.

When physical love reaches a refined level of exchange through polarity, love is generated as a tangible reality between a man and a woman. In being profoundly touched, woman connects with the source of her own love and showers man with her love, thereby completing the circuit of love and joy. Remember again and again: any level of awareness brought into sex will begin to create love; it is the awareness itself that transforms sex into love. Once again, it is not what we do but how we do it. Woman is love, this is the quintessence of her very soul; thus, love to her is as essential as food. She requires the opportunity to relax into her feminine nature and receive the contentment and regeneration of ecstatic experiences to sustain her life. The sincerity and willingness of both parties is clearly a contributing factor, but the responsibility also lies in the individual's hands. Through cooperation in sex we can regain power and balance as male and female forces.

Tantric Inspiration

There is certainly something very similar in very different emotions: the overwhelmingness. It may be love, it may be hate, it may be anger—it can be anything. If it is too much then it gives you a sense of being overwhelmed by something. Even pain and suffering can create the same experience, but overwhelmingness has no value in itself. It simply shows you are an emotional being. This is typically the indication of an emotional personality. When it is anger, it is all anger. And when it is love, it is all love. It almost becomes drunk with the emotion, blind. And whatever action comes out of it is wrong. Even if it is overwhelming love, the action that will come out of it is not going to be right.

Reduced to its base, whenever you are overwhelmed by any emotion you lose all reason, you lose all sensitivity, you lose your heart in it. It becomes almost like a dark cloud in which you are lost. Then whatever you do is going to be wrong. Love is not to be a part of your emotions. Ordinarily that's what people think and experience, but anything overwhelming is very unstable. It comes like a wind and passes by, leaving you behind, empty, shattered, in sadness and in sorrow.

According to those who know man's whole being—his mind, his heart, and his being—love has to be an expression of your being, not an emotion. Emotion is very fragile, very changing. One moment it seems that is all. Another moment, you are simply empty. So the first thing to do is take love out of this crowd of overwhelming emotions.

Love is not overwhelming. On the contrary, love is a tremendous insight, clarity, sensitivity, awareness. But that kind of love rarely exists, because very few people ever reach to their being.

Osho, transcribed teachings,
Om Shantih Shantih Shantih

PERSONAL SHARING

Tantric Sex Completely Changed My Life

It is unbelievable how much has changed in the past months since the "Making Love" retreat. When I think about what has happened to me, tears start running and I am infinitely grateful for these experiences and for this gift in my life. Again and again, I am confused and I keep thinking: "This can't be true. I am for sure on some sort of trip." But the trip does not seem to end. For the very first time in my life, I realize that I have treated my body badly and that I can stop this without effort from one moment to the other. The physical symptoms that come up are so strong that the beautiful sensation of having an orgasm is nothing compared to it. It is good to know the price I pay for a beautiful orgasm, and that I have the choice to pay it or not. Usually I do not feel like being totally worn out for two or three days due to having had an orgasm. So many big and small things have happened that I have for sure forgotten some of them.

Most importantly, my partner and I have come closer than ever before. Emotional moments have become more and more rare. We love to spend very, very much time with each other and have a hard time not being in each other's presence. That has been different in the past. We had moved into a bigger flat just because we could not stand living together without each of us having a room of our own. Now we have reorganized the flat and the single rooms have become a shared bedroom and office. This way we can always be in each other's presence and feel the love flowing back and forth.

My encounters with people are different. My heart is open. In the past I took a long time to develop trust in someone. This now happens much more swiftly. My connections are less language-oriented. I don't like talking as much as I did; I prefer to be simply here, feeling inside of me and perceiving what is happening. A lot of talking is strenuous for me and takes me away from myself. Whenever I used to meet a woman, an inner movie was going on: "We could have sex with each other. Do I want her? Does she want sex with me? But I have a girlfriend. Bummer!" Now when I meet a woman I feel that my heart is open, that everything is okay, that I can talk with her and feel good. I have no need for sex as my imagination used to suggest. I encounter the person in a way that has not been possible for me before. I really see her, instead of avoiding her in a way. Of course this does not always happen, but more and more often.

In the morning my lover and I both do our t'ai chi and other morning exercises together. This gives me pleasure and I'm amazed how much it helps me to stay grounded in some critical moments. My need for a career, money, fame, appreciation, exciting journeys, and meeting many friends has faded. I prefer to be with my beloved and am very content with that. If I could change my life from one day to the next, I would love to have work that allows me to stay at home every day, and not travel around all the time. Recently we were apart for ten days, and I easily lose the connection to my heart when I am alone. In the past I always wanted to be at home in order to come close to myself.

In the last month I woke up twice because I had an orgasm. I did not ejaculate. I had not experienced that since puberty. For one of these incidents I had a dream with wild sex fantasies. We have short moments with a hot kiss, but the desire for hot sex is there for only a second and vanishes before we have time to put it into practice.

I realized that my lust for sex has evolved into lust for life. Sometimes so much joy is bubbling up in both of us that we feel like exploding. My woman's menstruation is now normal, as it had not been for a very long time, and she has normal ovulation again. I can hardly believe my life has changed so much in such a short time and in such a soft and harmonious manner. Thanks a lot.

PERSONAL SHARING
Staying Connected

With tantra I often realized how my love has the effect of my going beyond myself. The union of vagina and penis is firm as a rock, which keeps reminding me of my love. As waves of hate or fear threatened to deluge me, that connection helped me to stay aware of my love. With the help of love I would then share my fear, as opposed to being trapped in it and projecting it onto my wife; as we all know, the projection of fear is the most wonderful fertilizer for fights and separations. Overall, tantra has helped me to deal with my patterns and fears. I can stay much more grounded when a pattern comes up, and name the pattern. Once it's out in the open on the table or in the bed, I can more easily deal with it constructively.

Tantric Inspiration

When you come back after a Tantric sex act, you have risen, not fallen. You feel filled with energy, more vital, more alive, radiant. And that ecstasy will last for hours, even for days. It depends how deeply you were in it. If you move into it, sooner or later you will realize that ejaculation is a waste of energy. No need of it—unless you need children. And with a Tantric sex experience you will feel a deep relaxation the whole day. One Tantric sex experience and even for days you will feel relaxed—at ease, at home, nonviolent, non-angry, non-depressed. And this type of person is never a danger for others. If he can, he will help others to be happy. If he cannot, at least he will not make anyone unhappy.

Osho, transcribed teachings,
Vigyan Bhairav Tantra

10

PERSONAL EXPERIENCES

In the pages ahead you'll find a small selection of the numerous letters we have received from men and women over the past years. We can attest to the authenticity of all these letters, which are anonymous for reasons of privacy.

LETTER SHARING (MAN)
My Penis Touched Her Heart

Two weeks after the wonderful retreat, we are still deeply touched by our new experience of making love. It seems like a miracle that our relationship could change in such a fundamental way after thirty years. We could never imagine that our problems in coming together—our different ideas and expectations of having sex   would find a solution in this new, conscious, and very simple way of making love. And we are fully aware that this solution is not simply the end of an old problem, but much more the beginning of a new way of making love on a totally different level. It is a spiritual practice that leads us to our true nature, and which is able to heal us and heal the world.

Every time we feel my penis being attracted by her vagina, it is magic. We never imagined that a man's penis could immediately touch the heart of the woman. We feel the energy flowing—deep joy, peace, and love. It is a kind of coming home, of relaxing, and of pure existence. We will never forget these moments; they have already begun to change our lives. Before it was unimaginable that we would come together every day. Now we are not only enjoying our daily "quickie," but usually we also make love in the evening, in a more intense way. We both feel there is something missing when we don't come together and connect.

We both know that we are at the beginning of a long journey, and we want to continue.

LETTER SHARING (MAN)
Enjoying the Landscape

I'd like to share a picture that came into my mind: Conventional sex is like mountain climbing, straight up to the peak. Tantric sex as I learned it with other "neo-tantric" teachers is still like climbing mountains, reaching for higher peaks than in conventional sex, and then dancing for a while near the peak until you reach it.

Tantric sex, as I learned it with you, also happens in the beautiful mountain landscape. But long before you start getting exhausted by climbing to the peak, you find that there are lovely meadows, marvelous forests, small brooks with clear water you can drink . . . so you just start walking around the mountain. From time to time you can see the peak, or climb to it whenever you want, but usually there is no need to, because it is so beautiful where you are.

LETTER SHARING (MAN)
Feeling Places I Did Not Know I Could Feel

I started my career as a sexual being at age twelve. It happened during a birthday party, and although (to be honest) it was a quite short experi-

ence, it became the blueprint for almost the next thirty years of sex. All I wanted was to get back to the feelings I had when that girl touched me and let me inside her.

Needless to say, I never felt that way again. But I tried everything. And so I started traveling to some really strange places on my roadmap to fulfillment. I did things I would now like to undo, and I used some people who really loved me. I felt myself drifting away from what I was looking for, and the more I drifted, the more I fought to cling to it. In the end, I fought so hard I could not remember what it was. To cut a long story short, by the time I got to your retreat for the first time, I and my sexuality were full of disappointment, anger, and tons of aggression. By then I thought it had to be that way.

I could not imagine sex without moving, licking, and so on. No wonder I felt slightly uncomfortable when you told us about a kind of sex that included none of this. It was difficult to deal with strange things like meditation, finding a home inside myself, or massaging the perineum, but nothing was comparable to my panic when my penis was inside my wife and I had no idea what was going to happen next. The panic reached all-time highs when my penis started to shrink while inside my wife. I felt lost and powerless, as if my penis were no longer a part of me. All the anger and frustration stored inside of me turned into a huge wave, ready to drown me. There was just one solution: movement, friction, and ejaculation. Welcome, black hole.

Gradually, with the relaxation of a week of meditation, I became more and more aware of myself. I felt touches in places where I did not know I could feel anything. In fact, it was new to me to be touched without getting aggressive or horny. It was such a relief to just lie down and listen to my body. I started to feel excitement all over my body, not only inside my penis. The speed of lovemaking slowed down day by day. My body experienced that orgasm and ejaculation are not the *same. Sometimes they were, but even the feeling of ejaculation changed. Good-bye, black hole.*

When I came back from the week with you, I came back with the feeling that I had forgotten something really essential. All the ghosts of the past came back, and this time, hitting the floor really hurt. Once again I lost connection to myself, and no bodywork or meditation could bring me back home. We returned to your retreat to listen to you both one more time. I don't know what happened and I don't want to know what happened, but somebody or something brought us together again. There's just one word for it—grace. I'm really grateful and I hope I won't spoil it again this time.

Believe it or not, it took me four weeks to write these few sentences. If it had been a letter instead of an e-mail, there would be tear stains on it. Thank you for being not teachers, but two human beings who live what they preach. You have a place in my heart forever.

LETTER SHARING (MAN)
The Rewards of Being Present

My wife and I attended your "Making Love" course this year and completely changed our style of sex. We decided that sex has to have high priority in our lives. We make three or four appointments for making love on weekends, and two or three during the week. And in the morning we often do exercises; I like to stretch my body and get a feeling of my perinium and pelvic floor area. It is beautiful to be connected to my wife and closer through making love. We have less stress and tension around sex since we began practicing cool sex. And we laugh more while making love, for example when we change position. For me it is good that my wife always feels my penis. There is only one condition: To be present. I think my challenge is to be present and to learn to talk about my feelings.

LETTER SHARING (MAN)
Postmenopause Miracle

Since we'd been working on ourselves for more than twenty-five years and giving mental training seminars for three years, we had the feeling we knew at least the tip of the iceberg, yet you taught us much, much more.

For the past ten years, since the changes due to menopause, we had given up sexuality, but we are now living what we both call a "wonder" or a "miracle." All the doctors and the few trainer/teachers we had approached confirmed that in nature, "Women are, in fact, old models," and that we would have to live with this situation. I adjusted, but fortunately, my wife did not give up. She had the feeling that despite not being fond of sex, something was missing in our marital partnership.

Since we met you on the first night of the "Making Love" seminar, and after our very difficult and depressing experience on the following afternoon, we began making love two to three times a day with utmost pleasure and love. Although all the doctors (including a gynecologist) told us that the dry, closed, and painful vagina could only be reactivated with the help of regular hormone therapy, which my wife did not want at all, things have actually worked out to be as they were in our very young days. She is smooth and lubricated, and with love and pleasure as never before, not even at age twenty-five. For us this is a wonder. And with this completion of the circle, the love, tenderness, pleasure, care, ease, and happiness that has entered our partnership is at its very best. Nobody knows how happy we are, except us, of course.

With the easy way things are going now, we both believe your words—that this world can live in peace and happiness. We are spreading the word and hope that eventually it will reach all humans, and that all those who can see and feel the truth will live a new life with joy.

LETTER SHARING (MAN)
Making Appointments for Lovemaking

First, thank you once again for the beautiful week. It was a milestone in my personal journey toward myself. Now, after a week of practicing what we learned from you during the retreat, I notice that I feel completely different—calm, present, happy, and content—and many tensions have disappeared. Although my everyday life continues to have many obligations, I am going through it more serenely and without hurry.

The fact that I have dropped the very idea of goals in lovemaking gives me a totally different feeling in my body, mind, and emotions. Now I know that I don't need to go anywhere or do anything, but just feel and rest in the present moment. This gives me enormous trust in myself and in life, because now I know that I don't need to create anything and that I just have to wait for things to happen on their own. Also, the fact that my wife and I make appointments to make love is a totally different approach in our relationship, because knowing that we both are willing to go forward in lovemaking makes me satisfied and without anxiety. I don't need to wonder whether she wants to be with me or not; I know she wants! And this is such a relaxing feeling.

All of your "Love Keys" are so important: eye contact, slow penetration, breathing, heart opening, and so on. But one of the most important things is that lovemaking becomes like a continuous exploration, because so many things are coming to the surface. Sometimes we don't know what is going on—misunderstandings also arise—but at the end the sky becomes clear and serene and we have new insights. In any case we feel closer to each other and more loving. Of course we have just opened this door a little, and we know that we have just a little experience of what we have learned from you, but it seems like a new page in our lives.

LETTER SHARING (WIFE OF THE ABOVE MAN)
Healing Hatred toward Men

I would like to add a few things important to me. In our lovemaking many of my old fears, distrust, and anger toward men came out. It was sometimes very difficult for me to accept all my old hatred toward men, but I managed it, seeing that my husband is not that kind of man at this moment. He is full of love and compassion, and that helps me a lot. But also after those difficult moments, today we had some wonderful experiences. Feeling his penis inside, doing nothing, was such a tremendous joy, I felt that now life is beautiful, and it just goes on and on. It is some kind of miracle for me, and I thank you for that.

For me it's sometimes difficult to look at all the things that are coming up, to accept that lovemaking is like meditation, and to just watch what is coming up and not do something about it. But I like this process very much and see that I can become more aware through it, so it feels right for me.

LETTER SHARING (MAN)
Our Lovemaking Is Helping to Heal the Earth

Our lives have changed a lot in the past seven years, since we have changed a lot. We still pursue the same professions, own the same house, and so on, but within us something has changed considerably. We feel, sense, and see more, and most of all, we have learned to feel, sense, and see inside. In our daily encounters we reach physical, mental, and spiritual depths that we never considered possible.

Our love journeys have diversified. They lead us deep into our bodies, to Mother Earth, through space, to the sun, through the chakras and their colors, to temples, angels, and through previous lives. On physical, mental, and spiritual levels we are creating healing connections for our own healing and for the healing of others. We are sending healing energies to the earth, to war zones and disaster areas. We are breaking patterns from our past and from past lives.

We do all this in a deep loving connection, feeling the golden ring that streams from the penis to the breasts through the vagina, the garden of love, the kundalini line, and the organs. This golden ring stays with us throughout our everyday life. It also streams when we are not actually physically connected. It streams across continents, and we can sense our love connection physically when we are apart.

This ring, which we forged in our first tantra course, gets stronger and stronger, and we realize that the people around us can feel it, even if they know nothing about our tantric connection. We relate differently to life; we're more awake, more conscious.

Due to our healing connection we can participate in world affairs on a spiritual level, and we sense that it makes a difference. Our tantric connections are evolving. We feel this again and again with great pleasure.

LETTER SHARING (MAN)
Gratefully Relieved of a Job

I am writing to express gratitude for the beautiful and profound retreat that my woman and I attended in December 2008. For forty years I have been searching, researching, and experimenting, knowing deep down that lovemaking holds the key to the expression of love between a man and a woman. This search led me to tantra fifteen years ago, and with each workshop since, with some of the best teachers in the Western world, I ended up with just another set of techniques that focused on achieving various phenomena. Little did I realize that each of these was distracting me from what I wanted most, namely, to connect in love with my lover. What I learned in the "Making Love" retreat is that this is totally available for me in stillness in lovemaking. When my mind and body are still my heart opens and my penis becomes a vehicle of loving, healing male energy.

Also during the retreat I experienced what I can only describe as a change in consciousness around my male sexuality. Like all men that I know, since my earliest sexual experiences I felt driven by some force within me toward sexual pleasure and ejaculation. While I love sex and sexual pleasure, every so often I noticed this feeling of being out of control, as if sex had control of me. After my first tantra workshops and reading Taoist books on sex, I began to practice ejaculation control in lovemaking and conserving vital energy by not ejaculating with every experience of lovemaking. While this provided great sexual experiences and gave me the beginnings of a sense of mastery, it was still control of a strong biological urge and suppressing the habit of the intense pleasure of ejaculation.

During the "Making Love" retreat there was a shift. In our lovemaking we had the time to really experience what it was like not to move toward excitement. It was as if we created the space for something new to manifest. We had the opportunity to really appreciate one another. We experienced healing of past sexual hurts. We expressed the love that we felt. We saw and felt the beauty of male and female body joined in love. For me it was as if this deep experience of extended presence in love outweighed the fleeting pleasure of ejaculation.

There is a very practical aspect that I enjoy about this way of making love. In past lovemaking I always felt as if I had a big job to do. The first thing I had to do was to gently seduce my lover to get her interested in having sex, and then help her to awaken sexually so that she was ready for intercourse. The next part of the job was to build the level of excitement till she was approaching her orgasm. If I decided that I would ejaculate it was preferable that we try to orgasm together. Alternatively, I would have the job of withholding the energy and semen of ejaculation while she had her orgasm. That's a lot of work for a man to do. It didn't leave much time for me to experience and express love.

Now it's simple. Together we both look for the next opportunity to make love. We connect in cool pleasure and I have no job to do other than be present.

LETTER SHARING (MAN)
Opening and Closing My Heart

I will not give my power, my life-power away again. Since the workshop I feel alive, my heart is beating strongly. I am full of beans. I feel grateful for my love, my cheerfulness, my joy about a new day and about this gift. But I also feel pain for the many times when I did not, or could not, do what I actually wanted to do. A kiss with my beloved in the morning, a loving embrace, looking into each other's eyes, and sharing joy about life and about this moment cause me to laugh and cry simultaneously. It is coming from a deep place. I feel it streaming through my heart as it opens and laughs, closes down, and starts to cry.

Now I am sitting here and my heart is wide open, and in this moment I feel in touch with the silence, the joy, the love. Here, I also feel like opening and sharing it. Slowly the pain about things I did not do, about the love that was not expressed, dissolves. Yes, I am bringing light into the darkness, into the fear, and it is disappearing. Now I also understand that you can show me the way, but I have to walk it. Yes, I am walking, and sensing, and enjoying. Life is so beautiful and I am a part of it.

LETTER SHARING (MAN)
Finding a Deeper Connection

The days with you have been a refinement for us on all levels. Our lovemaking has become slower, more energetic, and less athletic. I did not have any physical discomfort with conventional sex, but often felt energetic conflict before, during, and after the sex, which had led to weird moodiness.

Now that we have become more conscious and slow, I feel more bal-

anced, ever more often finding that relaxed, flowing, powerful quality of being that I have always looked for on other paths, but never found so easily and naturally. In our hearts we are more deeply and softly connected with each other, while on the level of personality there is more space between us, which reduces the emotions.

LETTER SHARING (WOMAN)
Making Time for Breasts

Over Christmas and New Years we had a difficult time. I was not really centered and our old issues about closeness and distance resurfaced. Many emotions came up and it was not easy to get out of them. We had a shift and then we had an extra long, very relaxing time. Tantra has become a familiar form of lovemaking, and for me it is a beautiful key to come into my body, open up, and connect. If we succeed in meeting in the cool love-zone and really drop into it and connect there, I feel very nourished on a deep level and I am in bliss.

I experience our encounters as always different and sometimes very intense. I feel a lot and I've ridden the waves of energy. And then sometimes it is totally different, subtle, and relaxed. I feel very clearly how my body responds, opens, and relaxes on a cellular level, and sometimes this happens when we are simply connected, as if that is the call for relaxation. Hot love is still an issue, and if I succeed in engaging with it, staying in contact with myself, my energy, and mostly with my heart, I do enjoy this as well. The afterward time is our teacher, a beautiful experience.

I am just reading your book for women and I thank you here for it. It is really good to get background information that relates to my experiences, or to let myself be inspired by the exercises and explore them. I'm giving more attention to my breasts and I'm very happy to experiment alone with myself or during lovemaking. I have made extra time in my calendar for my breasts, and I want to deepen the connection.

LETTER SHARING (MAN)
Happy to Be Present

It was a revelation for me to finally find out how I can integrate spirituality in my relationship and my sexuality, and thereby heal myself and my partner.

I feel as if I arrive much more at home, and as if I found my true calling: to learn and live playfully and joyfully, and to share how we love and find fulfillment on Earth, thereby overcoming separation and freeing ourselves from the illusion of the ego.

It was an important part of my healing to watch how loving and respectful you two are with each other. Since I originally come from a family within which an extreme amount of fighting went on, it was very healing to see how love and respect can be practiced between a man and a woman, if we learn to understand our deeper essence. My relationship has become much deeper and more fulfilling. I am free of performance pressure and happy to see and live my part as a man—to be present.

PERSONAL SHARING (WOMAN)
You Have to Make a Lot of Love

I keep remembering your advice. When I said good-bye I was in great fear that at home everything would be different, and that all our problems would come up again. You felt my fear and said, "You have to make a lot of love." I did so, and something wonderful happened. My husband is more loving, mellower, and more tender in his whole being. The wrinkles in his face have disappeared and his skin is very soft. I believe that he let go of his difficult upbringing and conditioning during that week. I am very grateful that you guided us on this beautiful and sunny path. That's exactly what we have been looking for after our thirty-nine years of marriage.

PERSONAL SHARING (MAN)
The Bliss of Full-body Orgasm

For our love session (during the seminar) we retreated to our bungalow, which helped us to explore a totally new and healing closeness, and a new expression of our love. Since the beginning of the seminar we had been in close contact with our emotions and feelings, and we felt much more porous and sensitive than before the course. After a shower we cuddled and rested for about twenty minutes in deep relaxation. We looked long and deeply into each other's eyes. Then we put ourselves in the scissors position and connected without having an erection, and without feeling any lust.

We closed our eyes and took a deep breath in the direction of our genitals, while each of us tuned in to the inner polarity—calmly, without expecting or intending anything. After a while my woman felt very fine, short pulses of lust. My soft penis started pulsing very softly in her vagina. We both did not move. As we looked into each other's eyes, I felt as if the energy circuit between us had completed. We felt a ball of energy in our genitals. I could not tell anymore where my being, my penis, stopped, and where she started. Penis and vagina felt like one shared whole, like pure energy. Warm waves were running through my body and I thought, "This is it what it means to melt into each other."

We sensed subtle energies pulling my penis deeper inside her. She felt soft and velvety, both of us pulsing softly with each other. My penis curled deeper and deeper into her vagina, without my moving at all. We both experienced a new feeling of closeness, silence, peace, bliss, and lust at the same time. Her vagina had received my penis fully. I felt like a welcome guest in her, and realized how my penis had stiffened.

In this moment a wave of sadness rose in me. I had felt some sadness while we were making love in the days before, but this time the sadness was unbelievably strong and intense. Tears streamed steadily as I thought about what I had done with my penis up until then. It was so sad, so terrifying. All of a sudden I became painfully aware of all the unconscious sex with my woman and the women before her, how this had been caused by my goal-oriented behavior, and how the women might have felt with it. It is so painful to realize what mischief is caused by conventional sex. I had always considered myself to be a tender lover, but it is not the intention but the actual result that counts. My God, what have I done through unawareness?

It was as if I felt the pain of all women in my body. I am so sorry! I never intended that. I always intended to express my love. I simply cannot hurt the person that I love the most. While I was in tears and sharing all my insights with her, we were still united. Sobbing, I begged her to forgive each single moment in which I had been unconscious in sex with her. It was a relief when she said it had not been my fault, for it had happened without my knowing better.

Slowly I calmed down and began to feel a deep peace. I felt my heart from inside, and a connection between my base chakra and my heart chakra, which got more and more intense. My penis snaked again deep into her vagina. The intensity of the sex/heart chakra connection grew steadily, my breath got deeper, quicker, and stronger, and a powerful sensation of love rose up inside me. I stayed totally conscious with all that happened, more a watcher than an actor. I shared everything that happened with my woman. I felt how the energy in my penis started to rise inside of me. It was overwhelming. My penis and my pelvis filled with a warming energy, which finally streamed into the belly over the left side of my body up into my heart. My whole body was filled with the sensation that I usually have in my penis in moments of orgasmic ejaculation. The sensation went on and got more and more intense. It streamed into the left arm, down into the fingertips. It was overwhelming. On the left side of my body it continued streaming up to the place between my eyes. There seemed to be no end to it; it was a permanent feeling of ecstasy. All the energy had been streaming from my penis up into my whole body. Then my penis became soft without my ejaculating.

As previously experienced, I clearly sensed all my chakras as warming wheels turning slowly and continuously clockwise. It was a wonderful sensation. I laughed and had tears of joy, and had no idea how much time had passed. Finally, all over my body the sensation slowly faded, but in my heart I could still feel it for a long time. I was deeply satisfied. I had never experienced anything so beautiful in my whole life.

Later I asked my girlfriend what that might have been, and she said, "Darling, maybe you had a full-body orgasm."

Tantric Inspiration

The word *tantra* means the capacity of expansion, that which goes on expanding. Sex shrinks you, Tantra expands you. It is the same energy, but it takes a turn. It is no longer selfish, no longer self-centered. It starts spreading—it starts spreading to the whole existence. In sex, for a moment you can attain to the orgasm, and at a great cost. In Tantra you can live in the orgasm twenty-four hours a day, because your very energy becomes orgasmic. And your meeting is no longer with any individual person: your meeting is with the universe itself. You see a tree, you see a flower, you see a star, and there is something like orgasm happening.

OSHO, TRANSCRIBED TEACHINGS,
PHILOSOPHIA PERENNIS

EXERCISES FOR IMPROVING YOUR AWARENESS AND SENSITIVITY

Practice is the best way to improve in any area, and sex is no exception. There are a number of ways to "practice" awareness by yourself and develop sensitivity skills that will enrich your lovemaking. Familiarizing yourself with some of the sequences below will help you learn how to relax and engage your attention during lovemaking, so that you can be more fully present with your partner.

◯ Connecting with Your Own Body
Pulling Attention away from the Mind and into the Body

Becoming fully aware of your own body will make it easier to truly connect with another person's body, and this is easily done. As you sit or lie on your back you can start by closing your eyes and taking your attention to inside your body. As your awareness (attention) travels around the different parts of your body, discover a place within that feels good, restful, easy, a space that feels like home to you. This place can be anywhere below the head that helps you feel more rooted and anchored in your body, connected to it from the inside. If your whole body feels like home, this is fine, and if nowhere feels like home, this is also fine. The feeling of having a home within the body may become clearer in time, and if not, that's all right, too. This suggestion is only a tool, not a special technique.

Continue to rest and be with that part in your body, bringing awareness into the tissues. The inner realms of the body are also your flesh, guts, and marrow, and the source of your cellular aliveness. It takes practice to learn to identify and give value to finer bodily sensations, the delicious, subtle vibrations of life streaming and flowing through you. If you sincerely begin to love, honor, and pay attention to your body's inner world, it will soon become second nature. You can connect with your "inner home" at any moment of the day, while sitting, driving, eating, walking, or resting.

◆ Becoming Aware of Habitual Tensions
Relaxing the Body from Head to Toe

It is enormously helpful to scan the body and check for tension while you are making love. Or at any other time of the day. If you've never done this in an organized way before, it might be useful to practice on your own, perhaps as you're lying in bed preparing for sleep. You can also do this sitting or standing. Begin by becoming aware of each part of your body from head to toe, and relaxing each individual part. You will notice how the body takes a deep breath as you relax, letting go of subtle tensions. Allow each part to melt down into the part below it, until it all melts out the bottom of your feet. Your crown melts down into your forehead, which softens down into your eyes, and then into your cheekbones. This continues into the mouth and jaw, and on down into the shoulders, allowing them to drop down a few inches. Continue on down through your body, taking particular care with classic tension spots such as the solar plexus (take a deep and conscious breath here), let go of the belly, relax the buttocks, and release the anus.

Breathe gently and deeply through the diaphragm and into the belly, infusing the floor of the pelvis with vitality. Maintain awareness of your breathing whenever possible and for as long as possible. Whenever you find your attention drifting, shift back to your own body and breath. Keep scanning upward and downward and notice where (and how easily) habitual tensions reassert themselves, and relax! Make scanning and consciously relaxing tense parts an ongoing process. Notice how every "let go" is usually followed by a sense of inner cellular expansion. Men report that consciously relaxing the anus and buttocks repeatedly while making love reduces the pressure to ejaculate. More "space" is created internally, and the life force is able to circulate and expand through the rest of the body.

⬡ Position for Rest and Relaxation

Aligning Your Spine for Presence, Awareness, and Sensitivity

The ideal horizontal position for relaxation is with the head, neck, and spine aligned in one straight line, not even a few millimeters out of alignment, and with the head centered and not rolled to one side. Your legs should be straight and slightly apart, and the ankles should *not* be crossed. Place a narrow, soft pillow (or rolled blanket) *directly under* the crease behind the knees to create a slight curving and softening of the knee joint. Place a flat, firm, small pillow (or folded towel) under your head. Tuck your chin to your chest and straighten your neck before placing the pillow in position. The pillow should support the lengthening stretch of your spine so there is not too much of a curve in the neck. If the chin is pointing almost directly upward and not tilted toward the chest, use a slightly deeper pillow (or give the towel another fold) to lift the head an additional few inches and create length, which reduces the curve in the neck and brings the level of the chin down. Place your open hands palm down on the groin area, on either side of your pubic bone. Allow your breathing to become deep and slow. Scan the body and relax tensions. Rest quietly with your eyes softly closed for at least twenty minutes, holding awareness in your body generally, or in the home in your body as discovered in the first exercise.

⬡ Tantric Meditation
Peace Pervading Armpits

Lie in a relaxed position, as suggested in the alignment exercise above, for twenty minutes or more. Close your eyes, taking your awareness into your body. Start just between the two armpits and with your total attention "pervade an area between the armpits into great peace." Forget your whole body; remember the heart area between the two armpits and your chest, and feel it filled with great peace. When the body is more relaxed, peace automatically happens in your heart; it becomes more silent and harmonious. Done frequently, this practice will establish peace within you and make you feel more independent, and love will be more of a giving; you'll have so much peace, you'll want to share it. You will be returning to a source in yourself that is always there.

⬡ Extending Awareness of the Physical and Energetic Bodies
Tantric Meditation for Growing in Consciousness

As you lie in the aligned position already described, you can deepen your experience by closing your eyes and imagining yourself looking backward into your body. Imagine that vision is reversed and your eyes can look inward and downward into yourself, even as far as your genitals. Breathe deeply and slowly into your belly, as if the breath is massaging your insides and touching your genitals. Continually pull your attention back into your body and use the subtle sensations in it as an anchor. Deliberately disconnect from distracting thoughts when they pop into your mind. Let them float away, and instead return home and immerse yourself in the body so that you feel a sense of resting deep within. The sensation of being submerged in yourself. Travel with your awareness to any places in the body that are tingling, pleasant, alive, or warm, or where fine vibrations are present, and be with them, dissolve into them. Notice how inner sensations expand when you take the time to feel and acknowledge them.

At a certain point, once the practice of immersing into and merging with your senses takes root, the feeling of your having physical boundaries will disappear; you will feel as if you dissolve and become as light as a feather, bathed in golden light, floating suspended in the universe. You are, but you are not. In this way you can grow in consciousness until every cell is penetrated with light. The moment consciousness touches the cells, they are different. The very quality of the cells changes. Sensuality is gradually awakened as consciousness filters through the body.

You can set a clock alarm for the amount of time you wish to devote to the experience, or you may leave it up to your inner clock to spontaneously return you to normal consciousness, with the sense of having lost all track of time. You are likely to notice that afterward you feel refreshed and rejuvenated, as though you have had a drink directly from the source of life. It is also beneficial to practice this meditation before sleeping at night and at any time during the day when you need to recharge your energy.

◑ Awakening the Rod of Magnetism
Bringing Attention from the Head to the Perineum

This visualization will help you shift attention away from the head of the penis, where it goes automatically because it is there that intense pleasure is experienced. Envision your penis as a channel or conduit, and refocus your attention on the base of your penis, in the area of the perineum. The perineum, a small, coin-sized area of knotty muscle lying directly in front of the anus, is virtually the root of the penis and is its energetic source. It is where the muscles and tissues that form the penis initially emerge from your body. Begin to visualize your penis as a channel for potency, warmth, and love. Imagine it to be a wand or fountain of light and liquid gold that emanates from the perinium and streams along its length.

When you begin to make love and feel the heat rising, bring your attention to the perineum. Consciously relax the entire area, including the anus. When you notice your attention start to drift—there are, after all, abundant distractions—you may notice that the pelvic floor area once again contracts and tightens. Repeatedly relaxing the anus and maintaining awareness of the base, the perinium, will give you an inner feeling of your penis as a complete unit, rather than a disembodied tool for thrusting. It instead becomes a divine instrument capable of channeling subtle energies that flow or stream from the root upward to the radiant head and beyond into your receptive partner. Be aware of your breath and of the subtle sensations deep within your physical core as your inner rod of magnetism awakens. Notice how the life force rises to caress your heart into vibrant aliveness.

When you make love with your partner, take this awareness of the inner rod of magnetism with you and relax into the receptive containment of your partner's vagina, knowing that there is nothing to be done but relax and notice how energies awaken, flow, expand, simply because you put your attention there.

PERSONAL SHARING BY MAN

It is like a new beginning—a tentative and vulnerable new beginning. Getting to know both in theory and in experience that by placing awareness and presence inside my body, energies begin to flow, all by themselves, and that then can mingle with those of my partner. A very important shift was seeing my penis and my role as a male as being noble and that my "task" is to be fully present in my penis and ultimately deep in the vagina. Nothing more, and this is my deepest longing.

I feel, more than ever before, that I can direct my attention into my body, my home, my perineum. Especially honoring and focusing on my perineum gave me great joy when it responded by radiating beautiful energies. Overall this attention to my body, and the fact of doing more exercise, has allowed me to relax more deeply, calming my mind, releasing chronic restlessness.

I truly see this approach to the body and sex as the deepest form of peace work for the planet. Personally and collectively I see it absolutely necessary for healing.

RECOMMENDED BOOKS
AND RESOURCES

BOOKS AND RESOURCES
BY OSHO

The Book of Secrets. New York: St. Martin's Press, 1998.

My Way: The Way of the White Clouds. Pune, India: Rebel Publishing House, 1995.

Sex Matters: From Sex to Superconsciousness. New York: St. Martin's Press, 2003.

The Tantra Experience. Pune, India: Rebel Publishing House, 1998.

Tantra: The Supreme Understanding. Pune, India: Rebel Publishing House, 1998.

Tantric Transformation. Pune, India: Rebel Publishing House, 1998.

For more information about Osho and to purchase books and CDs, visit www.osho.com.

BOOKS AND RESOURCES
BY BARRY LONG

Love Brings All to Life. Audio CD

Making Love 1 & 2. Audio CD (Sexual Love the Divine Way)

Raising Children in Love, Justice, and Truth. London: Barry Long Books, 1998.

Stillness Is the Way. London: Barry Long Books, 1989. To purchase these products from Barry Long, visit www.barrylong.org.

BOOKS AND RESOURCES BY DIANA AND MICHAEL RICHARDSON

Richardson, Diana. *The Heart of Tantric Sex: A Unique Guide to Love and Sexual Fulfillment*. Alresford, Hant, U.K.: O Books, 2003. [Originally published by Thorsons/Element in 1999 as *The Love Keys: The Art of Ecstatic Sex*.]

——. *MaLua: Light Meditation for Women*. Guided breast meditation CD with music (English/German language). Cologne, Germany: Innenwelt Verlag, 2009.

——. *Tantric Love Letters*. Alresford, Hant, U.K.: O Books, 2011.

——. *Tantric Orgasm for Women*. Rochester, Vt.: Destiny Books, 2004.

——. *Slow Sex: Making Love a Meditation*. Rochester, Vt.: Destiny Books, 2011.

Richardson, Diana, and Michael Richardson. *Tantric Love: Feeling versus Emotion—Golden Rules to Make Love Easy*. Alresford, Hant, U.K.: O Books, 2009. [First published in German in 2006.]

To purchase books or CDs, visit www.livingloveshop.com. For further book information, visit www.love4couples.com or www.livinglove.com.

Translations of some books are available in German, Spanish, Swedish, French, Italian, and Chinese.

FURTHER RECOMMENDED READING

Robinson, Marnia. *Cupid's Poisoned Arrow: From Habit to Harmony in Sexual Relationships*. New York: Random House, 2009.

Rosenberg, Marshall. *Nonviolent Communication: A Language of Life.* Encinitas, Calif.: PuddleDancer, 2003.

Tolle, Eckhart. *A New Earth: Awakening to Your Life's Purpose.* New York: Penguin Books, 2006.

Zurhorst, Eva-Maria. *Love Yourself and It Doesn't Matter Who You Marry!* Carlsbad, Calif.: Hay House, 2007.

ABOUT THE AUTHORS

Diana Richardson was born in KwaZulu, South Africa. She holds a law degree (B.A.LL.B) from the University of Natal, Durban, South Africa, and has taught therapeutic massage since 1978. In 1979 she became a disciple of Indian mystic Osho and began a personal inquiry into tantra—the union of sex and meditation—inspired by Osho and tantric master Barry Long.

Through the integration of these different sources in her own experience, a unique body of work on "generative sex," or "cool sex," has emerged, which represents an evolutionary step for the human being. The essence of the teaching is encapsulated in the simple, practical, and highly effective "Love Keys." Since 1993 Diana has led "Making Love" seminars for couples with her partner, Michael Richardson.

Michael Richardson was born in Germany and attended the Academy of Music and Performing Arts in Stuttgart. He teaches tantra and t'ai chi—yang style as taught by Master Chu—as well as the Gurdjieff sacred dances, practices shiatsu, and is a musician. In 1985 he became a disciple of Indian mystic Osho. His thirty years experience of meditation in movement through the practice of t'ai chi planted the roots of his perception of energy within the tantric dimension.

Couples travel from different parts of the world to participate in Diana and Michael's informative and life-changing workshops in Switzerland. They are pioneers in the sphere of human sexuality and among today's leading authorities on the subject. They have published several books about the essence of tantra—the union of sex and meditation—and the practical ways a person can experience a more fulfilling love and life.

"MAKING LOVE"—A TANTRA MEDITATION RETREAT FOR COUPLES

The authors facilitate weeklong retreats in Switzerland and guide couples in the art of tantra. For more information on these retreats, please visit their websites listed below.

www.livinglove.com
www.love4couples.com

You may contact Diana and Michael by e-mail at the following address.

info@livinglove.com